natural
stress
and
anxiety
relief

Helen Johnson

Published by:
Helen E Johnson
Post Office Box 8058
Gold Coast Mail Centre
Bundall
Surfers Paradise
Queensland
Australia 9726

Tel: +61 (0) 7 55 275 225
Mobile +61 (0) 412 014 684

email: helen@johnsonstressrelief.com.au
www.johnsonstressrelief.com.au

First self published 1998, "Attacking Anxiety".
Then as "Stress & Anxiety". A Commonsense Approach to Treating Panic Attacks, Obesity, Depression and Chronic Fatigue Syndrome.
Published in Australia 2008 "Natural Stress and Anxiety Relief". How to use the Johnson Breathing Technique.

Copyright 2011 Helen Johnson ND

Author:	Johnson, Helen
Title:	Natural Stress and Anxiety Relief. How To Use The Johnson Breathing Technique.
Publisher:	Helen Johnson, Qld
ISBN	Self published
Subjects:	Breathing exercise for health Self care, Health, Mentoring
Dewy Number	N/A

Dedication

To my three sons David, Alistair, Richard Fielding and to my best friend Lorraine Winstanley thank you for being there, without your love and support this book could not have been written.

natural stress and anxiety relief

Acknowledgments

My thanks and appreciation I give to the following people: My Clients world wide - you know who you are. Without your input and confirmation about Chronic Fatigue Syndrome, Depression, stress, shock/trauma, panic, anxiety, weight gain and weight loss, I could not have put together the dynamics of the successful diagnosis and treatment about which I have written.

In memory of my Father, whom I believe suffered from the worst Anxiety Syndrome I have ever seen. He lost a man overboard off his ship in 1942, WWII – he was thirty-two and lived in fear of being called to a court martial until the day he died, in his seventies. I saw you all my life and never knew what was wrong until I suffered myself, and then I was driven to find an answer. Thank you for lighting the way.

For always being true to yourselves I thank my former husband Adrian Fielding, his late mother and his daughter (my step-daughter), Liesa Brennan.

A special thanks to my friends Lorraine Winstanley, Christine Shand, Margaret Gilmour and my son David Fielding, my life's journey would have been incomplete without you.

To those of you whose timing was perfect, you offered me help when I really needed it. Hedley Pardoe – the first reading, overview and original title. Faye Hill and Jean Howarth – formatting. Artist Christine Shand - your graphic sketches convey the message in the book. The book itself would not have seen the printing press if it had not been for both Judi Restom and her sister Beverley Ott who did the editing and, Jean Howarth and Lynn Richards for enhancing my computer skills. You worked a miracle, thank you all.

Contents

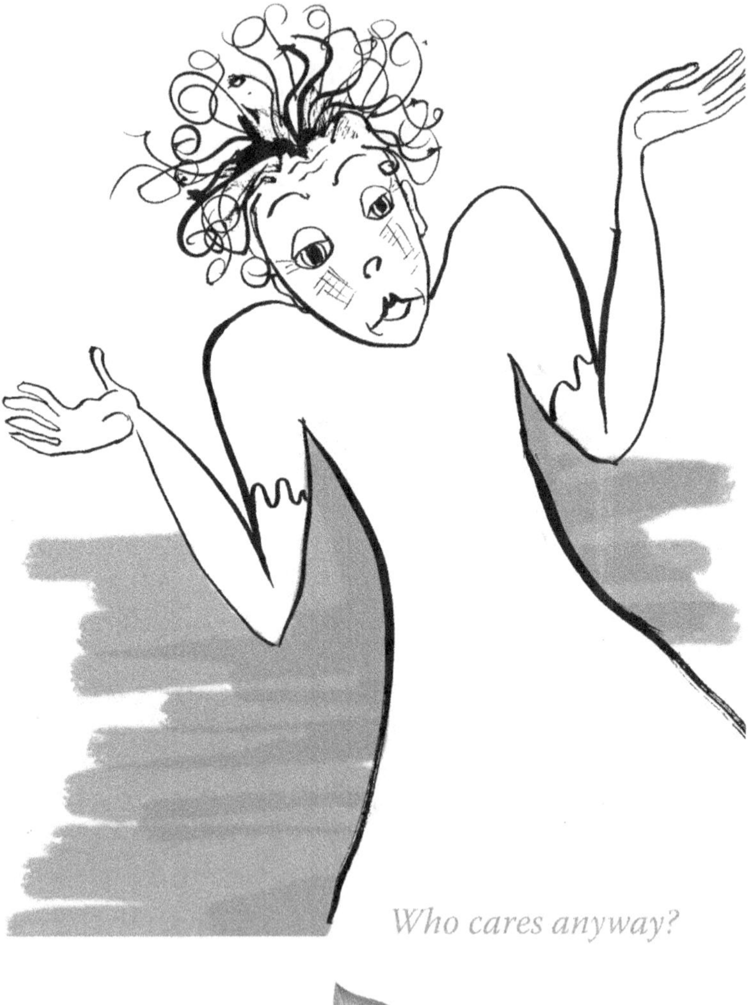

Who cares anyway?

Introduction

People are suffering. Stress is taking over. The body is becoming addicted to adrenaline. People all over the world are experiencing the disease symptoms associated with prolonged stress, shock/trauma and adrenaline.

Multiple Anxiety Disorders (M.A.D.) or Anxiety Syndrome is the result.

Do you know what it feels like to feel stressed and anxious?

Stress has many different ways of manifesting itself within the physical body and within the mind, and the various forms of stress and trauma that we absorb on a daily basis affect us mentally, physically and emotionally.

> **❝ ... stress and trauma are the tools we unconsciously use to put the body into panic. ❞**

Simply speaking, stress and trauma are the tools we unconsciously use to put the body into panic. And, simply speaking, by using the respiratory muscles correctly we can 'technically' stop stress and adrenaline from taking over our lives. However, having a friend and/or counsellor listen to us and really hear what we are saying also helps.

Stress is all about adrenaline – the fight, flight and fright, freeze response. To make the body experience these responses we unconsciously continually alter the way the respiratory muscles work when breathing. If we practice this often enough we learn a bad habit and cause the body to become addicted to adrenaline. We cause our own panic, stress and anxiety and we, therefore, can do something about it ourselves.

Adrenaline can be good and bad, what we need to do is identify whether the adrenaline response is creating normal or abnormal responses in our minds and bodies and learn how to, as a year twelve student said to me, 'harness the energy'. Stress and, therefore, adrenaline affects nearly everyone I meet.

To assess yourself, identify from my story whether you suffer from any of the symptoms. If you do, try the Johnson (Breathing) Technique, because, used properly on a daily basis it will give you more control over your life. By calming yourself you will help yourself learn to relax and improve your lifestyle and, if you practice the Technique before going to sleep, you will have a more restful sleep.

What a time I have had getting this down on paper. Over the past few months, every conceivable thing that could have gone wrong has gone wrong. Well, at least Murphy's Law survived!

Two computers have broken down - never to be repaired.

It is Christmas and there has been a huge family fight.

As soon as money comes in for me to spend on the things I need to enable me to write this book, another, even bigger bill comes in, demanding payment yesterday! I will not have the money until tomorrow and by then who knows what else I will need to spend it on.

The steering on my car needs fixing, the oil light is staying on too long, a squeak has developed in the action of the clutch pedal, and the gear lever needs new brushes (or something?), so that it doesn't vibrate when I drive for any length of time.

Do I sound stressed? The answer is, YES!

I suffered under the umbrella of Multiple Anxiety Disorders for many years. These disorders were an ever increasing, often-repeated pattern in my life and you will notice that at times my writing style also reflects this repetitive pattern.

Is there chaos in some area of your life? Can you also relate to repetitive patterns in your life? Is this a recurring scenario for you as well? Does stress trigger your anxiety?

If so, then read on, because I have found that no matter what stressed and anxious people choose to do, need to do or have to do, everyone and everything around them seems to be there to stop them from doing it. So much so, that they never get their needs met. Instead, they end up feeling used, neglected, rejected, not noticed, depressed and worthless. Worst of all they feel lonely, alone and totally frustrated.

Family, and to a lesser extent friends, are the worst offenders. Why would they allow you to change anything? They have a vested interest in keeping you where you are. They need to keep you where you are so that you can keep on meeting their needs. And even though you are exhausted from meeting their needs, you still cling to your motto of 'peace at all cost' - and the cost is you!

It does not matter how much determination you have, how much you push yourself, how hard you try, how stressed you become, and how much panic breathing you do - breathing shallow, high in your chest, or taking big deep breaths, yawning and sighing, nothing ever changes because the stress of changing takes too much effort and once again you give in. Why? It is easier to give in than to fight for what you want and you ask yourself - who cares anyway?

You have been repeating the same old pattern for so long that you are now feeling too tired, exhausted and too depressed to bother changing anything. You can see that the whole system of effective living is collapsing around you and you cannot stop it.

People are becoming ill. Relationships, friendships and families are crumbling. You feel as though you are losing control. You can see that everything is out of control. You want to break the cycle and make changes, but you don't know how, you are just too stressed and exhausted.

The 'Technique' described in this book is not a miracle cure although it can be used by everyone - men, women and children. It has taken all of us a long time to get to where we are and it sometimes takes a long time to change. But, and this is a big but, it is up to you. With understanding, practice and persistence you can deal with your own stress, you will win out in the end.

There is something you can do to help yourself:

First, read my story and see if you identify with any of the mental, physical and emotional stress/anxiety symptoms, habits, patterns and behaviours. See if you can recognise some of the symptoms for yourself. Do they fit your profile or, perhaps, the profile of someone you know?

Second, understand the reasons why this happened to you and how you have kept the Syndrome going.

Third, learn to use the Johnson (Breathing) Technique at the end of the book. Harness your own adrenaline energy and control your own stress levels.

Who am I?

Obesity, stress, anxiety, fatigue, depression and panic are only some of the many adrenaline related symptoms I suffered from.

The **first half** of the book is my own story. It is sometimes repetitive so that those with the symptoms of stress and anxiety can identify themselves. It is about my search for an answer as to what was wrong with me and why did I feel the way I did. I knew there was nothing wrong and yet there was something wrong. It explains the part shock/trauma and prolonged stress played in causing me to develop Anxiety Syndrome.

> " ... It explains the part shock/trauma and prolonged stress played in causing me to develop Anxiety. "

If you suffer from any of the symptoms mentioned I hope this knowledge will help you to identify for yourself your level of stress/anxiety. You too can ask yourself, 'how long have I suffered the after effects of shock and trauma and prolonged stress'? You can assess for yourself how much the Syndrome has affected your life.

The **second half** of the book explains what happens to the physical body when it is stressed and goes into panic without warning, how we keep this habit/pattern going and what we can do about it.

With understanding and knowledge and by using the Johnson (Breathing) Technique you too can change your life for the better, as I have done.

We were born using the respiratory (breathing) muscles correctly and I believe that everyone needs to technically breathe correctly on a daily basis. We were not made to run on adrenaline (fight or flight) all the time, when we do, we cause dysfunction in the body and mind and illness follows.

For twenty-five years I felt sick – gradually putting on more and more weight, I felt depressed, exhausted and generally as if I had no control over myself, or my life.

I went from one medical and non-medical doctor to another. I tried all forms of healing, went to University, Naturopathic school and read every book on every subject that I could lay my hands on. I never stopped looking for an answer as to what was wrong with me; I searched constantly for an answer as to why I felt the way I did.

I was married for some of that time, and the mother of three sons and one stepdaughter. However, I never really felt happy or contented. I always felt exhausted and yes, I did get so ill in the end that I broke up my marriage and family, I even gave responsibility of the upbringing of our children to their father.

I thought that my children would be better off with their father because he was a good provider. I did not know how much longer I could keep going. I just did not have any energy left and I could not cope with the responsibility of rearing a family. Only people who have suffered at this terrifyingly low level will really understand how I felt. I felt as though I was no good to anyone especially my family.

In hindsight, isn't hindsight a wonderful thing? I now know that I was suffering from Anxiety Syndrome, an adrenaline addiction, and it was this that caused me to develop among other problems Chronic Fatigue Syndrome, severe panic attacks, Depression and huge weight fluctuations.

When I was married, for fourteen years our family was constantly on the move. We moved from one place to another within a state, from state to state within Australia and then from country to country. The shocks, both normal and traumatic, which I endured during that time, coupled with the constant unsettling stress of moving, gradually turned me into a permanently anxious person.

One of our moves took us to Singapore. Within four days my anxiety surfaced again and I took myself off to the doctor.

After much 'too-ing and fro-ing', asking and answering questions and many blood tests etc. he said to me, "I do not know what is wrong with you, but if you stay here you will die". He also added that he had sent another patient back to Canada with a similar problem.

He really cared about me and wished that he could help, but he did not know what was wrong with me.

And so we returned to Australia. My husband gave up a perfectly good career, more stress, and we bought a health food shop.

At that time I knew very little about alternative medicine - herbs, homeopathy, nutrition or remedial therapies (massage), but the seed was sown and much later I decided to study and become a Naturopath.

This decision came about as the end result of my life's situation at the time, rather than from choice. I was not fulfilling a great dream but doing something for the sake of appearances. If I appeared to be doing something worthwhile then everyone would leave me alone and I would have time to find out what was wrong with me. I hoped!

By now I was eating incorrectly, putting on weight, short of breath and puffing every time I did any exercise such as walking up a short flight of stairs. I always felt as if I could not get enough oxygen into my system and I felt as though I needed to take bigger and deeper breaths all the time. I was forever yawning and sighing.

I thought that if I did a course of study I could exert my brain energy rather than my physical body energy, of which I had none, and maybe I would start to improve. Studying was an acceptable behaviour and a good way to hide from everyone what was really happening to me.

> **"I sometimes wonder if there is a sort of chaotic order in the Universe, ..."**

I sometimes wonder if there is a sort of chaotic order in the Universe, because, when I look back over the years and assess the choices I did make, becoming a Naturopath was the only choice I had if I wanted to find out what was wrong with me. It was all about timing. At the time there was no University in my area, becoming a Naturopath was my only option. Now there are two universities, Bond University and Griffith University.

Any other path would not have forced me to search in the directions in which I did to find the answers to the questions I was always asking myself and everyone else, "why am I so tired and why do I feel so depressed?"

My background and my upbringing were both traditional and conservative. The innuendo was always that a university degree was the only way to go. This for me, however, was not to be. I started and tried to finish a university degree many times, about five times I think, but without success. I loved studying and did very well writing

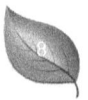

assignments but blacked out and suffered major anxiety and panic attacks when I was put under pressure doing examinations, which, of course, are part of every university degree.

I thought that I wanted to be a counsellor or psychologist and my direction at university had always taken me into the humanities, whereas, I really needed to be studying the sciences. However, as fortune, or is it fate, would have it, each time I settled down into the course I had chosen, a major trauma would occur, either for me or someone in my family, my anxiety would shoot through the roof, and I would give up University.

However, it was not only my difficulty doing examinations that made me give up I would also have a really good reason for giving up. This is a procrastination pattern that is also part of the pattern of anxiety.

Being able to follow through on a commitment is one of the hardest things to do for a person with an anxiety disorder. They, and others around them, put so much pressure on themselves to succeed after so many failures, that their nervous systems just do not cope they begin to experience burnout and, finally, either run out of steam or run away and have to give up.

Most of us who suffer from anxiety do not want to give up and fail. We are determined not to fail completely in life if we can help it and, it was this determination that pushed me into Naturopathy.

This time I did not fail. I finished the course and graduated. However, by the time the graduation night came along I had another huge realisation - there was no one there for me.

What a shock! Struggling to survive and having to deal alone with my own terrible feelings of loss, grief, guilt, shame and pain, because of my broken marriage, had isolated me from everyone. I had been struggling so single-mindedly to survive and keep going after losing my home and family that I had forgotten to include others in my life and I could not think of anyone who would be proud of me and like to come to my graduation so I did not ask anyone.

I can remember standing there, in my pink cocktail dress with my hair too short, looking out over the crowd of happy people, feeling totally alone and detached from everyone. As I was being presented with my Diploma, I thought, "what price success? What is life really all about anyway?"

I felt isolated from the fun everyone else was sharing but unbeknown to me changes were on the way!

Naturopathy had opened up a whole new world for me. I was propelled forward into the fields of study that would eventually give me the answers I was looking for.

As a Naturopath I studied many different subjects, including anatomy and physiology and, eventually after years of searching, I came to understand the devastating effect that prolonged stress and shock and trauma can have on the nervous system and therefore, on our lives.

Gradually I began to understand how human beings can develop and suffer from multiple anxiety disorders, Anxiety Syndrome, and how they keep the Syndrome going in themselves. Finally, twenty-five years later, after much soul searching, questioning and analysing, I stumbled upon a way of controlling my stress and, therefore, my own Multiple Anxiety Disorders.

At first there was no joy, only hard work mentally and physically in trying to understand what was happening inside my physical body when I practised the Technique I had found.

Gradually I realised, however, that I had something that was working for me and slowly and surely peace, healing and an unusual feeling of control began to return to my life. There had been and still were many triggers in my life which caused my problems. I had practiced for many years to be the way I was and it took some time and many ups and downs before I did finally understand and reverse the process.

For years I had been questioning myself. What was wrong with me? Why did I feel so tired? Why was I always out of breath, huffing, puffing and breathing high and shallow in my chest? Why wouldn't my mind stop racing and give me some rest? Why did my decisions always seem to be the wrong ones?

Why was I suffering so much pain throughout my body - neck, shoulders and lower back? Why was I overwhelmed by, and wallowing in, so much emotional pain - feelings of loss, hurt, rejection, anger, low self-esteem and low self worth?

By nature, I really am a very positive person but what was this cycle I was in, and how could I break it?

Why couldn't I feel, act, and behave in the positive and productive ways that I perceived others did?

Other people made right decisions in their lives. They appeared to lead successful goal oriented lives and achieved what they set out to do, but not me? Why?

I always felt disconnected from others, as though there was something missing, something wrong with me. I thought that I projected an image to others of being motivated and positive and perfectly in control on the outside, even though on the inside I felt out of control. This, however, was an illusion on my part. I have since been told that I projected quite the opposite image.

Denial is a big issue for anxious people. Stress/anxiety affects nearly everyone to a greater or lesser extent and we know it but we cannot stop it, so we try to ignore it. But it doesn't go away.

We do not see ourselves as others see us. We do not know how hard we are to live with. We think prevention is better than cure and that keeps us very busy. And, if we are not always busy then we are usually the opposite, asleep – very frustrating to live with. Others do notice, begin to wonder about us, move away from and us leave us feeling even more anxious and lonely than before.

My mind was on automatic. It just would not stop thinking and worrying unnecessarily. I could not sleep. My fears were running at an all time high and my adrenaline activated nervous system was going flat-out, systematically sensitising and conditioning itself into automatically manifesting all the symptoms and characteristics of what I now know to be those which are associated with Anxiety Syndrome.

I was living in fear. I began to fear fear itself, the more frightened I became the worse I felt. I withdrew further and further into myself and away from other people, and always with legitimate excuses.

I tried to hide how I was feeling from everyone. I would think, there is nothing wrong with me but there is something wrong with me. I felt so confused and frustrated.

Experience had taught me to stop talking about myself, because no one really wanted to listen to me or understand how I was feeling. I tried to explain to everyone what was happening to me mentally, physically and emotionally but no one wanted to hear me. They were all thinking, and some even said to me - "pull yourself together there is nothing wrong, just get on with it, (life)".

I spiralled down again and again into defeat. I was very depressed. I could not understand why I was suffering so much. Was there no answer? And still I kept smiling, covering up, trying to hide what was happening to me. The more I tried to hide it, the more tired I became.

Feeling this way caused me to be forever on the move. I did not want to 'feel' or 'think' anymore. Others drink, drug or medicate to get away from their feelings and thoughts, I just kept on moving restlessly around.

Even though I was on my own and always tired, I moved from house to house. I never stayed at home I kept on pushing myself.

I visited people and wandered around shopping centres, stopping to look in the shops that interested me, dress shops, bookshops, antique shops, etc. Then one day at my lowest point I walked into one of our local bookshops and found exactly what I was really looking for.

I was standing aimlessly looking at the books in the healing section when a man pushed past me and knocked a book off the shelf onto my right foot.

> " ... Then one day at my lowest point I walked into one of our local bookshops and found exactly what I was really looking for. "

I picked the book up to put it back on the shelf. As I did so, I casually looked at it and saw that it was a book about nervous problems.

As I looked around I saw other books on the same subject, so I decided to have a look at them and found, at last, a few pointers about what was wrong with me.

I stood there in stunned amazement with the gradual realisation that my problems were physical they were coming from my nervous system. The thought that I had a nervous disorder had never entered my head. I had always thought that my problems were psychological, in my mind, something to do with past unresolved mental/emotional issues. But surprise, surprise, I had been looking in the wrong places.

This time, in my excitement, I didn't panic breathe, I just plain forgot to breathe and nearly choked in the process.

At last I had something to identify with. I was so overwhelmed with relief that I burst out crying right there and then in the bookshop and, for once I did not care.

As I thought about myself over the next few weeks and read a few more books on nervous problems, I realised that my problems were not in my mind. I was not going mad, crazy or insane. I was not manic-depressive, or having a mental breakdown and, most important of all, I was not losing control - what a relief.

I knew for the first time in years that I was not having a stroke, a heart attack or dying - my secret family fears.

Gradually I came to understand what was wrong with me. My nervous system was out of control. It was spontaneously putting itself into panic, without any conscious directions from me.

At last I could stop searching for what was wrong with me. I could also stop blaming myself and others for what was happening to me.

My nervous system was running on adrenaline and going into panic all on its own and manifesting all the symptoms of Anxiety Syndrome, I had no control over *it*. In fact, *it* was controlling my life. No wonder I always felt as though I was not in control. Why was this happening, I asked myself?

With a sudden flash of insight I realised that all internal systems, organs and glands inside the physical body - digestive, reproductive, respiratory (breathing), circulatory (beating heart), nervous, immune, endocrine, lymphatic and metabolism, etc., are part of the sub-conscious system.

The sub-conscious system responds instinctively and automatically to what? It cannot be influenced by the conscious mind. It does not make decisions or respond to any decisions made by the conscious mind. So what does happen?

This system has a mind of its own and is on automatic all the time. It functions independently of the conscious mind, as does any other habit or pattern, such as writing or spontaneous panic which is conditioned into the sub conscious system.

Now the questions really started. If this was a habit I had programmed into my sub-conscious system, how was I going to get rid of it from that system? What was I going to do about this? How was I going to stop this happening? Was there a cure, and if there was a cure where could I find it?

Having kept my nervous system under prolonged stress for many years and, by exposing it to one shock after another, I had systematically sensitised it to automatically and spontaneously respond to any form of stress or shock triggers by manifesting one, many, or all of the symptoms and characteristics of Anxiety Syndrome.

By responding in the way that I did to life's experiences I had systematically taught my nervous system to behave the way it did. The consequences of this were enormous. I had, through the lifestyle I was living caused my own problems. I had done this to myself. The original triggers no longer existed I, however, was keeping this habit going myself. I had been practising for many years to perfect what I was doing. But what was *it*, what was I doing?

I felt both devastated and elated. Devastated because my life was in ruins, but elated because if I had caused this damage to myself, and my lifestyle, then there was a hope that I could 'undo' the damage. I knew that I could not give back to myself the lifestyle that I had lost, but maybe, I could give myself a better quality of life from here on.

Suddenly there was a light at the end of the tunnel.

I knew what was wrong with me, and for the first time in years my anxiety symptoms began to lessen, my Depression hesitantly lifted, my weight began to go down, all on its own, and I felt the stirrings of freedom, joy and happiness within me again. These were amazing feelings. I had forgotten what it felt like to feel good.

I also noticed that for once the black cloud, that surrounded me and in which I lived, had dispersed and in its place everything seemed to be lighter and brighter.

I wanted to share my excitement and happiness with someone, preferably my family, but there was no one left to share with. Both my nuclear and extended families had turned their collective backs on me and disappeared out of my life. I was still in touch with them but at a distance.

> " They were fed up with trying to keep up with my every move. They stopped listening years before ... "

They were fed up with trying to keep up with my every move. They stopped listening years before because a Psychiatrist suggested to a male member of my family that I had a mental illness. They believed him and dropped me, I did not realise this had happened until much later. This type of collusion between authority figures in our lives, where the label 'mental illness' is concerned, causes so much emotional damage to the victims and, except for a few very close friends, who could see the real 'me' past the label, there was no one I could turn to.

I took a good long look at my life and down I went again. I felt so alone and was totally overwhelmed by feelings of loss, rejection, grief, guilt and every other negative feeling that you can name. I spiralled

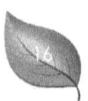

down into an even deeper blacker, lonelier depression than I had ever experienced.

I had no concrete identity. No familiar sign posts to hang on to. No family - my children were in the care of their father. No home of my own - the court had authorised that I sell our home and contents when we separated. I was no longer a married woman with a partner and family.

I was now a single woman who needed to relearn the rules of survival alone. For someone with Anxiety Syndrome who already lives inside a dark cloud of depression, feeling as though they are both haunted by and disconnected from everyone, this situation appears to be insurmountable.

Having already made the decision to withdraw from society to 'find' myself, I was now living in a comfort zone, which I had created for myself, one I controlled. Here I was safe, and the fear of stepping out again into the big wide world on my own was totally terrifying.

I had stopped weaving the normal cycles of life into the fabric that is life itself. The greatest grief of all was that I could never look forward to those family gatherings, which traditionally families share - births, deaths and marriages. They were lost to me forever - I had to weave a new fabric - alone.

I can remember when I was a child sitting in Church one Sunday listening to a story about Jesus Christ, I heard that Jesus made a difference for the better in many peoples lives and I foolishly thought, as children do, that maybe one day I could make a difference, for the better, in the lives of other people.

However, quite the opposite was happening. I always set my goals but I just could not achieve what I wanted to achieve, the harder I tried to help myself and others, the worse the havoc and destruction around me seemed to become, especially for me. I just could not see my way clear to change anything for the better.

What a mess I had made of my life. It really was not my fault. It was situational. My nervous system, which is part of the subconscious system, just did what it wanted when it wanted and took me with it. I was later to realise that shock/trauma and prolonged stress were my triggers; they kept me in this state.

My negative thinking continued and, instead of wanting to live and make a 'difference' in the world and in other people's lives, I actually began to nurture a hope that the end of my journey was near. I wished, at night, that I could just lie down, go to sleep and never wake up again. I, personally, never thought about suiciding, however, I thought at times it might be an easy way out. Anxious people think about everything – even suicide.

Clinical experience early in my career:

When I was first started teaching this Technique to clients a married couple came to see me. The husband was very stressed and anxious and had been for many years.

About forty-five minutes into the session I realised his wife had not said a single word. Just as I noticed this she burst out crying. She sobbed and sobbed and as her sobbing stopped she looked up at both of us - her husband, who was looking absolutely amazed, and me, sitting there in shock wondering what I had done to cause this reaction – and said, "if we had met you four months ago, my nephew would be alive today. He was suffering from everything you are talking about. He committed suicide three months ago.

He was seventeen." I felt so sorry for her and wished that I had been able to help, because, I too had suffered and knew some of what he must have gone through before he died.

The session was successful the husband responded well and was grateful for the help, although, all of us were a bit subdued after his wife's revelation.

Having spoken to many people over the years, I now think that Anxiety Syndrome may be one of the causes of youth suicides. If I am right there are many young people who can be helped.

Most of what was happening to me I hid from other people and, as one of my clients once said to me, "we become good actors when we have this Syndrome, don't we?"

My answer was an emphatic, 'yes'. We are always wearing a mask and hiding from others what is happening inside us, because they don't understand us any more than we understand ourselves. When I eventually understood what was wrong with me, I felt a great sense

> " ... We are always wearing a mask and hiding from others what is happening inside us, ... "

of relief and some of the tension flowed out of me. Even though I still wanted to hide from myself and everyone else, this feeling of relief was different it was tinged with something else, hope maybe?

I believe there is a natural survival instinct in all of us and, it is this instinct that begins to surface. Otherwise, why do we struggle against all odds to keep going?

There was light at the end of the tunnel and it was growing brighter as I moved closer to my answer. I kept thinking to myself, I know what is wrong so there must be a treatment, or hopefully a cure and on I pushed, searching, searching.

Gradually my depression lifted. At last I had a mission, a reason for living. I knew what was wrong with me and now I wanted to be well. For the first time there was one thing I did know, my symptoms were not controlled by my mind. My mind could not and did not control what was happening to me, therefore, my reasoning told me that the symptoms were related to my physical body and the conditioning therein. Both my mind and my body were, thanks to adrenaline and the nervous system, running too fast. All I needed was a way of stopping this happening. I needed to find a treatment and hopefully a cure.

It was about now that my life began to change.

notes

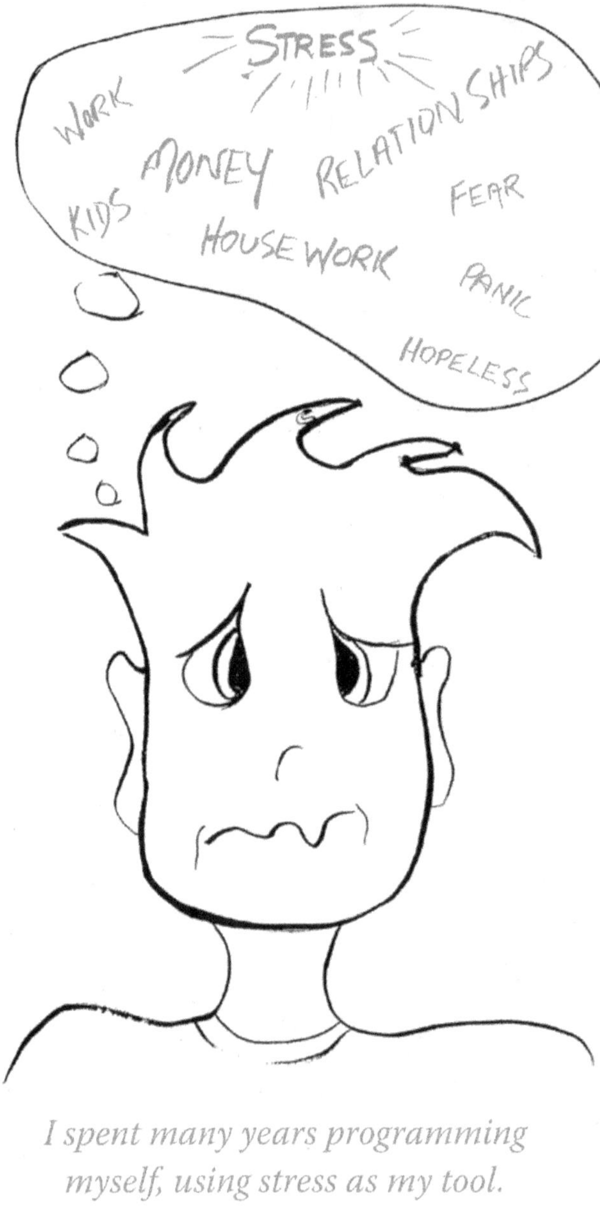

*I spent many years programming
myself, using stress as my tool.*

What happened, what followed?

I am a naturally healthy, strong and resilient person. However, without knowing what was happening to me and as I look back over the years, I can see that I spent many years programming myself using stress as my tool, into my own Anxiety Syndrome. But, how did I do this?

I had actually sabotaged myself with my own strength. The more I hurried to keep meeting deadlines, the worse my stress symptoms became. The more the perfectionist in me struggled to do everything perfectly, the worse my symptoms and the Syndrome became. My conscious thinking mind kept pushing me to perform but physically I was getting weaker every day. Emotionally, I felt very weak and vulnerable.

> " ... The more I hurried to keep meeting deadlines, the worse my stress symptoms became. "

I would cry anytime - in a sad movie, if I thought of my children, saw them or heard anything about them, I would cry for no reason at all. I missed my extended and nuclear families and cried over them - I cried about everyone and everything.

I had progressed from bouts of acute fatigue into chronic fatigue, feeling aches and pains all over my body all the time. All I wanted to do was sleep, especially in the daytime, I was putting on weight,

I was eating the wrong foods (sugar) and my digestive system was playing up - wind, bloating and burning, constipation or diarrhoea. I thought food was the cause of these problems, it was not.

At night I could not sleep. My mind was on automatic and would not let me sleep. I would lie there for hours on end thinking and worrying. My negative, slightly hysterical self-talk nearly drove me mad.

All through this time I experienced, with prolonged stress, a number of major shocks and traumas. This put my nervous system under even more pressure and I became so sensitised to feeling anxious that the various symptoms associated with anxiety were there all the time. By now, I was really exhausted.

How was I to help myself and make a difference in the lives of others?

I was now beginning to feel as though I really could not have cared less, but life has a way of playing tricks on one. Slowly and surely, as I withdrew from my responsibilities and the people and situations around me, my survival instinct came to the fore. Thanks to my Naturopathic training, and my naturally curious mind I began to understand what had happened to me.

There are three ways in which anxiety disorders of the nervous system can develop: prolonged stress, shock and trauma, and a combination of both prolonged stress and shock/trauma.

What is prolonged stress?

Prolonged stress has many triggers - work, money, relationships, etc.

Ask yourself. Do you handle these issues easily and successfully, or do you feel upset, stressed and worried by them and the effect they are having on your life? Have your attitudes and behaviours changed in any way to accommodate stress?

Example 1

Does driving to work upset you? Is it the road rage of others or is it your own road rage you cannot handle?

At work is it your boss or your workload that you cannot handle? Do you have to much work to do and not enough time to do it in? Do you feel angry and take your frustrations out on yourself and others?

Is there someone at work with whom you clash? Someone who triggers your stress?

Does this person pick on you all the time? Do you pick on them? Does she/he know what they are doing, or not? Are they deliberately trying to upset you? Do they have an Anxiety Syndrome is it affecting their attitudes and behaviours?

Conversely, does your anxiety and fear stop you from standing up for yourself? Does your fear stop you from getting your needs met?

Does this type of situation make you want to retreat, give in and withdraw. Does the situation leave you feeling powerless, sick, tight in the stomach and nauseated? Do you dry-retch or vomit every time it happens? Can you feel yourself beginning to 'panic breathe'. As you breathe high and shallow in your chest, do you begin to feel weak and start trembling, or, defensive then aggressive? What are your reactions?

Example 2

Do you handle money well? Can the people around you handle money? Money issues can cause some of us more stress than anything else.

Example 3

Did you grow up in a family where you felt truly loved and secure, or did the opposite happen to you, did you feel as though your needs were never met, leaving you with residual feelings of anger, loss, rejection or abandonment?

Did you feel too protected, smothered, controlled? Were you not heard, not seen? Did you feel as though you didn't exist for 'them'? The more you tried to please 'them', the more they ignored you and your needs. Did this make you feel worse until eventually you rebelled from the sheer frustration of not getting the attention you needed.

As you grew up, did your feelings of anger/resentment/fear grow with you? Did you become sick? Did you begin to self medicate, e.g. sugar, junk food, cigarettes, drugs, alcohol, etc. Did you develop an addiction that made you feel better in the short term but, in the long term, made you feel even worse and more distressed?

Were you the sick one in a healthy family, so that you got all the attention, or were you the healthy one in a sick family so that you got none of the attention? Both of these patterns can suffocate the normal development of our instincts for healthy survival and leave us feeling anxious. Are your current relationships functional?

Do you feel as though other people are trying to control you? Are people always telling you that you are a 'control freak'? Do you need to be in control of everything so that you can keep the peace within yourself? Do you believe stubbornly that you are right and the rest of the world is wrong? Have you been called a control freak?

If you cannot get your own way, do you withdraw and blame others because they will not do it your way?

Another type of prolonged stress is the situation where couples, for months or even years, participate in the IVF program. This is both traumatic and stressful and, it could be that the high level of pressure they put themselves under to 'perform' is one of the reasons why conception does not happen. Why would the body procreate when all the signals are that it is in panic, fight or flight, i.e. survival mode?

The reproductive system is one system we have no natural control over so the alternative is to concentrate on the one system we can control, the nervous system and adrenaline. Use the Johnson (Breathing) Technique to release built up stress whilst you are undergoing the IVF programme. Help your own body to relax as much as you can.

Long term pain of any kind, e.g. back pain, causes prolonged stress.

All of the above situations, and many others, are situations in which prolonged stress can cause the slow and insidious development of Anxiety Syndrome.

When we live in fear or under stress for any length of time we alter our posture, pull our lower abdominal muscles in. This forces us to breathe high and/or shallow in our chests, causing the body to respond by going into panic, fight or flight.

Your level of debility, when this happens, depends on many things - what your stress is about, how long you have been stressed and whether you have been shocked and/or traumatised at the same time.

Shock/Trauma

Trauma follows shock. Shock is the initial reaction of a person to a suddenly life changing event and, although some people handle shock well, others do not.

Shock happens suddenly rather than over a long period of time and can be caused by such events as the premature birth of a first child, an ill child, a difficult birth, an operation, a car accident, your spouse walking in one day and saying that they are leaving you; finding out that you have cancer or diabetes; being told that you have to move, moving house within a district, state or country; moving schools; loss of a business, redundancy, bankruptcy, or even such simple things as being booked for speeding, can shock and traumatise a very sensitive person.

> **" Shock happens suddenly rather than over a long period of time and can be caused by ... "**

Suffering a deeper mental/physical/emotional shock, such as the sudden death of someone whom you loved dearly - a parent, spouse or child, can leave a person traumatised and suffering from the symptoms of multiple anxiety disorders for a very long time, sometimes for years after the event.

Any form of abuse causes the nervous system to go into shock – trauma follows. Physical abuse such as rape, incest, strangulation, beatings; mental abuse such as being always told you are stupid, worthless, brainless, of being ignored as if you do not have a brain and cannot think for yourself; or, emotional abuse, never having your emotional needs met or acknowledged does affect the nervous system. The after effects last for years because of the internalised associated emotions, e.g. fear, etc.

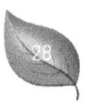

28

Shock/trauma and prolonged stress can be likened to cement. Cement takes years to cure that is set hard, and it has been suggested that shock/trauma 'cures' also. We need to acknowledge our shocks and traumas when they happen and do something about them. The nervous system internalises shock and trauma, therefore, using the Johnson (Breathing) Technique will help to settle the nervous system down. If nothing is done at the time of the shock, the 'curing', begins and the after effects reverberate throughout our lives sometimes for years. This is one positive way we can help ourselves.

If a domestic animal gets knocked over by a truck, it will run under the house as far away from we humans as it can until the shock subsides, then, when it has settled down it will come out from under the house wanting food and water, even if it has a broken leg. It looks at us as if there is something wrong with us because of the fuss we are making. It has forgotten by then that it had a shock and should be suffering the symptoms of trauma. Humans, however, do not forget.

Humans can only take so much. If they continue struggling to deal with their own thoughts and feelings alone whilst trying to take care of those nearest and dearest to them, they may get to a point where the pressure becomes so great that they explode.

After many years, the build up of pressure within me caused me to explode and I had to use that energy. At times my behaviour would be quite manic. Anything I set my mind to do in the short term I did faster and better than anyone else and no one could keep up with me. However, eventually the pressure of being manic exhausted me and I imploded.

From being an outgoing, fun loving, vivacious extrovert I became introverted. I withdrew from my responsibilities and became a self-centred person who analysed everyone and everything. I continued attending courses, reading and searching. I knew what was wrong but not how to treat it.

The books on nervous system disorders impacted me because I could identify with what the authors had written. Nearly every page described what was happening to my physical nervous system, but the biggest shock was still to come. At a later date I was absolutely amazed to find out that all of the physical, mental, and emotional symptoms and characteristics I was experiencing were actually classified as mental illnesses.

Can you imagine how frightened and angry I felt when I realised that a few health-care practitioners, some family members, friends and acquaintances generally believed that I suffered some form of mental illness?

There were times when my paranoia did take over. I thought that there were 'secret' things being said about me behind my back. I often felt as though I was not 'in' on discussions, particularly about me, and that others knew more about me than I did and maybe this was true at the time. There was collusion particularly between male authority figures in my life. However, I also now know that this type of thinking on my part is anxiety thinking, it can be controlled. I realised I could not control what others said about me, however, I did have the power to take some control over my own thoughts.

During those terrible years I knew of only three male 'authority' figures that were ethical, had integrity and really helped me. They knew the truth about my situation, I did not have to explain anything to them and I thank them - an accountant now in retirement, a wonderful Headmaster of a boy's school now retired and quite simply a neighbour who later became a good friend. Each offered me support, mostly advice from a male point of view.

These people were like water to a dying person in the desert. They knew the difference between good and bad behaviour and used the labels freely. They supported me because of their own understanding of themselves and others. I knew they understood no words were really needed. They were the sort of people whose actions followed their words. They were living proof of the saying, actions speak louder than words. They did not just stand back gossiping behind my back they offered to help and did so, their actions supported their words. Letting me know I was okay.

I would like to qualify what I have just written by saying that the reverse can also occur. Many other male and female clients of mine have been degraded by collusion. They too have had to put up with the fallout of innuendo (gossip) from so-called knowledgeable people in authority.

Thankfully, I was blissfully unaware of the fact that I might have multiple mental illnesses when I started to look for a way of curing myself. However, when I realised my problems were classified as 'mental illness' it did help me understand why I was generally misdiagnosed by health care practitioners. It also explained the behaviours and attitudes of some of the people nearest and dearest to me.

It helped me to understand why I was treated as if there was something wrong with me. I tried anti-depressants for three days and had a severe reaction. Fortunately, for me, I resisted self-medicating with any other chemical such as alcohol. I kept thinking that there had to be another way to stop me feeling the way I did.

I did not know anything about mental illness and my Naturopathic training did not cover the diagnosis and treatment of mental illness. Therefore, I did not look at myself in the way a person trained in understanding traditional anxiety would. I did not look at myself, or family members, and see mental illness of any kind.

However, I now understand that I, and others in my extended and nuclear families, have and do suffer from varying levels of Anxiety Syndrome. They too have their fears. They also have lived with prolonged stress and experienced shocks and traumas that have affected their nervous systems and their lives.

My ignorance of the understanding of anxiety being a mental illness gave me the freedom to focus only on the physical, mental and emotional anxiety symptoms I was experiencing and what was happening to my nervous system.

I knew that for me, even though my mind was involved and helped trigger some of my attacks, the symptoms I was experiencing were not mental. The only connection I could find between my mind and my physical symptoms was that as my mind raced so too did the symptoms in my physical body.

My concern, therefore, was with how my physical nervous system, (both mind and body), responded to stress and shock/trauma rather than how my mind worked. At the time, it did not occur to me that my mind played any major part in all of this and even now years later I know that it does not play any major part in causing these symptoms, it is the way that the nervous system responds to shock/trauma and prolonged stress. The adrenaline surge that does the damage.

All I wanted was to feel better. I did not want to feel sick, suffer migraines that only went away after I vomited, be constipated or have diarrhoea depending on my level of stress.

I no longer wanted to feel tired and exhausted. I'd had enough.

Everything concerning anxiety seems to work in extremes, for example, I always felt as if there was something wrong, and yet I knew that there was nothing wrong. In other words how can there be something wrong when there is nothing wrong. This 'circular' thinking plagued me, and caused me to become very self-centred.

I wanted to calm my mind, stop feeling depressed and chronically fatigued. I thought I was the only one this was happening to. I had no idea that what I was suffering from affected so many people.

Anxiety Syndrome is a worldwide problem. People have been and will be affected mentally, physically and emotionally by adrenaline related disorders until they are taught about the connection between these disorders and adrenaline.

Because, no one ever talked about problems like these, I thought I was the only one suffering. Perhaps, unlike me, others knew that anxiety was classified as a mental illness and did not want to be labelled 'mental' so they did not own up to it. I did not know until I suffered that this is a taboo subject, a never discussed subject, in the modern world.

> "Anxiety Syndrome is a worldwide problem. ..."

Many of my clients have said the same thing. No-one talked about these things and all agreed that stress is a major issue in their lives. Most of them can remember what level of stress or shock precipitated their Anxiety Syndrome. They too, thought they were the only ones suffering from these problems and, like me, most could remember better times when they had been functional and happy people.

Some, however, are able to admit that these symptoms have plagued them all their lives. They say that they have never been without some of the symptoms and, when questioned, most knew why.

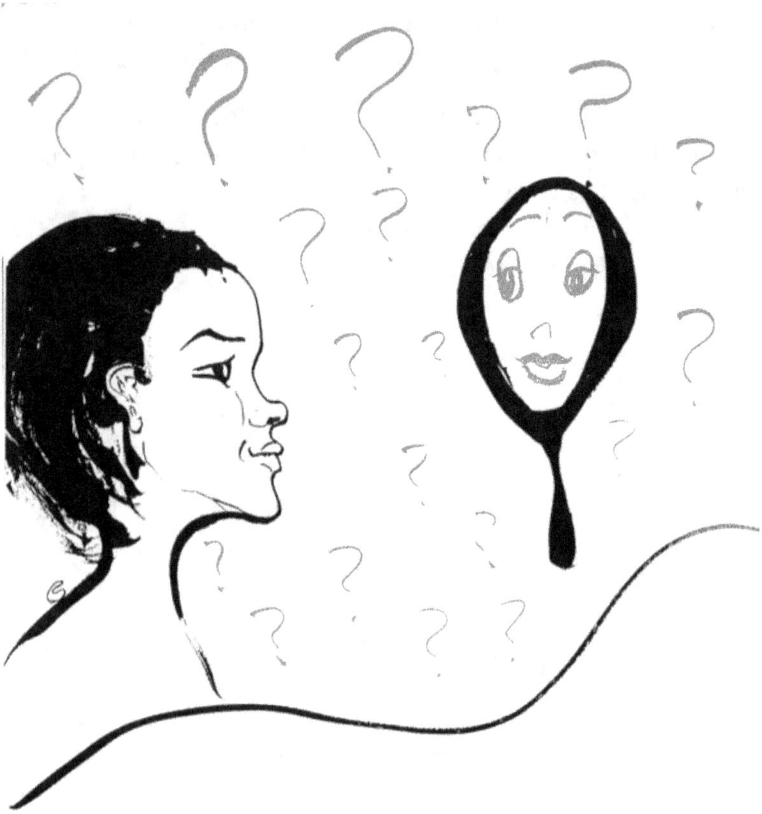

*Over and over again I asked
myself, what was I doing wrong?*

What is anxiety?

Anxiety is a feeling of unease. Anxiety symptoms are the mental, physical and emotional feelings, symptoms and sensations that are spontaneously felt throughout the body and mind when the nervous system spontaneously goes into panic.

There are three levels of panic – arousal, fight or flight and paranoia. The levels are reached and triggered by prolonged stress, shock/ trauma or by a combination of both and cause us to feel 'different'. We condition this response within ourselves by using the respiratory muscles incorrectly.

> " There are three levels of panic - arousal, flight or fight and paranoia... "

Continuing to experience stress, shocks and traumas we condition ourselves to spontaneously use the breathing muscles of the body the wrong way, this in turn locks in the 'different' feelings, symptoms and sensations until thought patterns, attitudes and behaviours change and sickness follows.

Why is this?

Very simply, there are two systems in the body. The Conscious or Voluntary Nervous System (the mind, the brain, the thinking system) which makes decisions about how we behave and live our lives, and, the Sub-conscious or Involuntary Nervous System which has under its control the habits/patterns and functions of all other internal systems, organs and glands of the body. Both systems work with one another.

The brain is the director. The Director decides to write a letter and sends a message to the conscious system to act, for example, pick up a pen in preparation for writing a letter. This we do consciously. After making the decision to write the letter, appropriate messages are automatically sent to the muscles of the subconscious system to spontaneously pick up the pen and start writing.

Simultaneously the sub-conscious mind responds to the command. This is a conditioned learned response that has gradually become an automatic response until we no longer have to learn how to pick up the pen and manoeuvre it to write, we just write automatically, we are thinking consciously only about the words we are writing not about how to manoeuvre the pen.

I believe it is this same conditioning that enables anxiety to take over our lives.

By responding in the same way physically to the experiences of stress and shock/trauma we cause the body to be flooded by many chemicals including adrenaline the panic hormone. This flood changes the way the body works. All the normal functions of the physical body are temporarily compromised when responding to the signals being sent to it.

How do we do this?

When we pull the abdominal muscles in we push the diaphragm up into the lung area automatically lifting the shoulders as we do so. It is this action that automatically triggers adrenaline. If we do this on a regular basis the body learns to run on adrenaline all the time, it becomes addicted to the chemical adrenaline and seeks more of it. This is an automatic response to stress and if we practice it often enough it becomes a habit which, like any other habit we cannot remove from the subconscious system unless we know first, what is happening and, second, what to do about it.

If we practice using stress, shock/trauma and the physical action of pulling the lower abdominal (respiratory) muscles in on a continual basis, we condition the sub-conscious nervous system to stay in a state of panic and, the physical body to become addicted to adrenaline. Therefore, because this system has a mind of its own and responds well to conditioning, with practice it becomes an ingrained habit gradually manifesting the characteristics and symptoms of Anxiety Syndrome automatically, and, all without any direction from the conscious mind. The conscious mind has nothing to do with this conditioning and neither do the lungs or the breath.

Breathing is altered only because of the action of the physical body. The action of the lower abdominal muscles on the diaphragm is technically the cause of releasing adrenaline and, therefore, the cause of Anxiety Syndrome.

Once this becomes a habit, it is no longer under the control of the conscious mind. The mind cannot control what is happening in the subconscious system. However, the conscious mind can control what the hands do, and it is possible to turn both the habit and therefore the addiction around by using the Johnson (Breathing) Technique.

Anxiety has many triggers both good and bad. Triggers such as danger, fear and happiness, all cause the body to manifest the adrenaline rush, the fight, flight and fright, freeze response.

How the body responds to these triggers is, from my experience, the cause of Anxiety Syndrome, and continually technically using the respiratory muscles incorrectly perpetuates the Syndrome. We breathe approximately fifteen times per minute. Correct diagnosis of all symptoms is the basis for treatment.

Consistently technically breathing the wrong way causes the body to learn a bad habit. We do not even know that we are doing this. We do not think about the way the body breathes.

> **"** ... using the respiratory muscles incorrectly perpetuates the Syndrome. **"**

When someone suffers a huge shock to the nervous system it becomes traumatised. The residual affect of this type of shock will be characterised by fear (panic) and, nightmares and/or flashbacks. These nightmares or flashbacks will often concern the traumatic event and can last for years after the event. This causes prolonged stress. Because of the breakdown of the body into physical/emotional/mental sicknesses we feel as though we have lost control over what is happening to us. This in turn causes feelings of fear. Fear, panic and panic breathing go hand in hand. Panic breathing drastically changes the functioning of the body.

Symptoms - Physical symptoms of adrenaline addiction

- Heart - palpitations or a pounding and rapid heartbeat. As a result of this increase blood pressure may rise. A feeling of pressure and pain in the chest or sometimes tightness

- Lungs - gasping for breath, sighing, breathing high or shallow in the chest with the feeling that you cannot get enough oxygen.

- Choking, coughing, wheezing, vomiting, shortness of breath

- stiffness, numbness and/or sometimes tingling in the hands and feet

- unsteady, shaking, trembling, and weakness felt inside the physical body

- shaking hands

- feeling dizzy, faint, foggy, cloudy, or like cotton wool

- major glands – swelling for no reason, immune system is not working efficiently

- feeling hot or cold, and flushed or freezing

- churning stomach, nausea, sometimes followed by spontaneous vomiting or diarrhoea

- to conserve energy there is a shutdown of non-essential operations like digestion

- secretions may alter, for example the mouth feels dry, salivation may increase

- excessive perspiration and sweaty palms and feet

- stomach - nausea, churning or upset in the stomach - wind, bloating and burning (acid, reflux) not enough digestive enzymes to break down food

- bowel/colon – diarrhoea is a nervous reaction

- constipation – the bowel/colon may appear to stop working properly for days, weeks or years because of shock and stress

- pancreas - a complete loss of energy throughout the body as the blood sugar level alters to deal with the situation

- some people develop a water addiction, they cannot stop drinking water and think that this is something to do with sugar diabetes, mostly it is not, however, a check with your local doctor for a diabetic test is a good idea

- Kidneys/bladder - for some, their usual urination pattern may change, urination may become more frequent. Fluid and swelling may appear in other parts of the body, for instance, around the ankles - especially with prolonged stress

- eyes - eyesight sometimes blurs other times becomes clearer

- muscles will alter their stress level to prepare for the fight or flight response - they will become tense and if they become tense often enough they will begin to ache and feel painful, cramps

- the blood sugar balance is altered spontaneously

- Adrenaline and other hormones flood the body. The gaseous exchange in the lungs alters releasing more oxygen into the blood and sometimes hyperventilation follows

- Feelings of being 'out of touch' with, 'dissociated from' or 'detached' from your body or your immediate surroundings.

Symptoms - Mental Thoughts linked to adrenaline addiction

- I cannot stop worrying and analysing. I worry about everything past, present, future and if there is nothing to worry about I will find something

- my mind/thoughts go around and around in circles

- I feel like screaming

- I'm going crazy, and having difficulty concentrating

- I must have cancer, or something very seriously wrong with me

- I feel like I'm losing control

- I'm going to collapse or faint or die

- I'm having a heart attack or stroke

- I must have a tumour on the brain

- I'm sure there is something wrong with my organs - heart or liver

- sleeping is a problem because my mind will not stop it goes on and on and keeps me awake

- I get a saying, song, or name stuck in my head and cannot let go

- I cannot stop counting.

Symptoms - Emotional feelings linked to adrenaline addiction

- depressed
- helpless
- shame/ashamed
- apprehension
- fear
- unadventurous
- distressed
- feeling irritable
- withdrawn
- frustrated
- forgetfulness
- worthless
- sad
- alone
- lonely
- terror
- desperate
- phobias
- listless
- loss
- on edge
- weak
- pain
- jealousy

- hopeless
- feeling like a failure
- tension
- caution
- constrained
- self-critical
- lost
- agitated
- restlessness
- clumsiness
- feelings of foreboding
- unhappy
- feeling sick
- empty
- crying
- tearful
- hate
- anger
- guilt
- overwhelming feelings of dread
- anxious/anxiety
- low self worth
- low self esteem

Symptoms – Behaviours and Attitudes linked to adrenaline

- All forms of abuse – mental, physical and emotional

- Suddenly losing ones temper

- Shouting

- Being overly possessive

- Aggression

- Rebelling

- Tantrums

- Head banging

- Arguing

- Always having the last word, verbally forcing others to give in

- Cannot sit or stand still for any length of time

I would like to point out here that some people will only experience one or two of the above symptoms, others will experience many of the above symptoms, and some experience all of them.

These symptoms are particularly overwhelming because of the adrenaline supported guilt/fear cycle that we self talk ourselves into, mainly because we do not know what is wrong with us. Expecting and waiting for something to happen sets the adrenaline off.

People easily lose confidence in themselves and withdraw socially. They fear making fools of themselves and their loved ones.

Then they start worrying. Worrying about everything past, present and what sort of disasters the future will bring.

Out of the chaos felt inside the physical body, ritualistic behaviours and attitudes such as the hygienically washing of hands over and over may start to appear. They have to return home to make sure the stove or the iron is turned off.

They cannot stop repetitive thought patterns and feel frightened, as if they are going crazy. They feel as though their minds are in control of them, instead of them being in control of their own thinking and thought patterns. Unbeknown to them fear is the driver and adrenaline the fuel.

Physically they continue to feel fear, breathe higher and shallower in the chest, lifting their shoulders as they do so. They pull all their lower respiratory abdominal muscles in, this pushes the diaphragm up under the ribs into the lung space preventing the lungs from breathing freely and it is this, often repeated, pattern that becomes the habit.

Obsessive Compulsive Disorders whether in behaviour, attitude or thought are very distressful and destructive to live with and may, in the long term, cause avoidance behaviour and Agoraphobia. Avoidance behaviour is most evident in those people who are locked in the house and avoid going out, even to go shopping. Many of them cannot go out they are too scared, fear and adrenaline have taken over.

Anxiety is the feeling of living in fear. It is the waiting for panic symptoms to happen. Panic itself is a cued or uncued response to people, situations and places. The more we practice panicking the more controlling are the various symptoms.

When I suffered from anxiety symptoms, I felt a complete mess and yet I struggled on until I became chronically fatigued. At one point in my life I would stay awake for only ten minutes then sleep for two hours or more. When I was awake I felt very depressed and guilty because I could not do anything other than take care of my own immediate needs.

For me this was a terrifying state of affairs. Previously I had led such an active life and the inactivity now forced upon me, nearly drove me crazy.

Around this time a dear friend took care of me. Without knowing what was wrong, she could see that I was withdrawing from my friends and family. I felt that they did not understand me. This in fact was the truth. They did not. She did not, but she cared anyway.

> " ... Previously I had led such an active life ... "

I did not understand what was happening to me.

Others could not understand why someone who looked so healthy and normal on the outside could not, for instance, go out and get full-time work or get on with life. They could not understand why I felt so depressed all the time.

Many clients have shared with me these same sentiments. They all knew that there was nothing wrong with their minds but they felt really depressed. They all agreed that suffering from chronic fatigue and the loss of their families and friends compounded their problems and made their anxiety symptoms/feelings worse.

This I know was not a mental Depression but rather a heavy overpowering feeling of being 'down'. At all times my conscious thinking was as rational and logical as it could be. If I was not sleeping or just too tired I could take care of myself and apart from the emotional help and support from my friend, I did take care of myself.

Even though my thoughts ran around and around in my mind, I knew that there was absolutely nothing wrong with my mind and its clarity. My problem was that my continuing analysis of my situation never gave me any peace, nor did it give me a satisfactory answer.

Over and over again I asked myself, what was I doing wrong? My mind never stopped asking questions. It just would not stop. A number of my clients can identify completely with these sentiments. They too, asked themselves and everyone around them, the same questions.

We nearly drove ourselves and everyone else around us crazy. The diagnosis, advice, treatments and theories were incorrect and our feelings of frustration grew alongside our symptoms of anxiety. The advice did not address what was really wrong and the treatments did not cure.

Often in Clinic, when I am explaining the theory to a client, spouses and partners, who have accompanied them, become very restless and sometimes quite angry. Their anger is not necessarily directed at their partners, but rather at continued misdiagnosis. Lack of information and incorrect diagnosis had, over many years, really interfered with their lives. All those years they were told that there was nothing wrong when, in fact, there was something wrong.

All because of misdiagnosis, anxiety had controlled and interfered with their lives. Many of them felt really angry because they could see exactly what they had missed out on.

When this happens I encourage both parties to understand that this Syndrome is not the fault of the person concerned, but rather it is situational. It is brought on by circumstances that are sometimes outside of the control of the individual.

I help them to understand that everyone handles stress differently and that no one is to blame. The nervous system, which is part of the sub-conscious system, just spontaneously goes into panic/anxiety when we are stressed and the conscious mind cannot stop it happening.

None of us realises that anxiety is situational, rather than deliberate, until we are told that it comes about because of the sometimes normal and, at other times, abnormal stresses of living.

The problem is that the individual may not cause or have any control over the situation that stresses them. They certainly do not have any control over the behaviour of the nervous system itself.

In other words, because we do not have any direct control over what is happening in the sub-conscious system of the body, we cannot, therefore, be blamed for developing Anxiety Syndrome. This is a great relief to most of us. We can stop feeling guilty about our past mistakes and get on with living in the here and now.

I explain to both clients and their partners that this Syndrome is insidious it just creeps up on us without any warning until we are debilitated by it in some way.

Most people know what the adrenaline rush is, and love the normal excitement associated with it, many, however, will deny the power of adrenaline as the cause of what is happening to them. Generally though, the client understands and accepts the theory, and agrees willingly to practice the Johnson (Breathing) Technique, assuring their partners that they are feeling much calmer after doing the exercise.

If clients or partners are in denial or sceptical of the treatment and want to argue, I suggest that they practice the technique anyway, even if it is to prove me wrong. I say to them - "stop thinking and analysing and do it anyway. This is a mechanical action directed by the conscious mind. Use your hands to make your physical body drop the adrenaline and feel what happens". Experience is a great teacher!

This challenge, from me, generally elicits laughter from both parties. The client is already beginning to calm down as the exercise takes effect and, it shows. She/he appears to be much happier and more relaxed and partners can see this.

The nervous system is the most powerful and important system in the body and if it is continually excited by stressful situations either good or bad, it becomes sensitised to excitement in any form and responds by releasing adrenaline.

> " The nervous system is the most powerful and important system in the body ... "

When adrenaline is released in response to excitement, either good or bad, every internal organ, gland and system changes to meet the need. Energy normally needed for other functions, e.g. digestion is diverted elsewhere, the metabolism slows down and we put on weight. Using the Technique correctly over two years brought my weight down by fifteen kilos, (30 pounds).

However, there is another reason why we gain weight. When the body is flooded with adrenaline, it (the body) shortly afterwards releases the hormone cortisol. This hormone is sometimes called the hunger hormone and is released to encourage the body to eat to replace energy expended when the body is stressed, i.e. after the adrenaline rush.

This becomes a catch twenty-two, an ongoing cycle, one follows the other.

If the body is stressed and runs on adrenaline it will automatically be driven to eat to replace its lost energy and, apart from dieting and exercising, the only way I know of changing this pattern of eating all the time to replace lost energy is to de-stress the body by dropping the adrenaline. Diet and exercise will not be effective unless adrenaline is under control. We can all lose weight under pressure, diet or exercise, but will it stay off?

Last year, 2005, I ran a six-week weight loss control program. All participants had not been able to break through their weight barrier and lose more weight. They knew about diet, had been to and tried every weight loss program available, they knew how to exercise but they did not know how to drop the adrenaline, stop releasing cortisol and reactivate the metabolism and digestive system.

I did not ask them to change anything except technically the way the body works when breathing. I taught them the Johnson (Breathing) Technique. At first they lost size, then weight. It worked for everyone. They were very happy with the results and most have kept the weight off. One said to me guiltily, when she came in to see me about a year later, "it's obvious that I have not been doing the breathing". She had put on weight.

Therefore, when treating any form of disease, including weight loss and/or gain, we need to pay attention to the nervous system. The nervous system is the most important system in the body it must settle down first before the rest of the body will respond to treatment on a long-term basis. Client history and correct diagnosis of what is really happening for them, is particularly important especially when a client has a history of shock/trauma and prolonged stress.

If treating the anxiety symptoms only, for a short time better health will be achieved, however, optimum health will not be held unless the nervous system functions correctly.

To understand how prolonged stress and shock/trauma affect the body, imagine a scenario where you step out onto a road with the intention of crossing it. As you step out, you see a truck speeding towards you. You are directly in front of it, so that if you stay where you are you will be run down.

Your instant reaction will be one of panic – fight or flight, and you will jump out of the way of the vehicle.

As you see what is about to happen to you, your conscious mind sends a message to the body telling it to save you from imminent danger. Your response is that you take a big breath and jump out of the way. You pull your abdominal muscles in and lift your shoulders as you spontaneously jump. When you are safely out of danger you relax your muscles and drop your shoulders, your whole body registers a feeling of relief, it relaxes and your bodily functions return to normal.

This is a natural survival response. However, what happens inside the physical body in those few seconds is critical to understanding this theory and why the treatment works.

As the 'jumping' individual takes a deep breath, the gaseous exchange in the lungs alters and more oxygen is released into the blood; simultaneously adrenaline is released into the blood and the blood rushes to the extremities (the head (brain), arms and legs), to enable the person to spontaneously jump out of the way of the danger.

What has happened to the body? In answer to the danger signal, the nervous system has gone into panic. It is responding to the survival instinct. This is a normal response to danger.

However, if we spend our whole lives responding to stress by panic breathing then effectively we are being chased by a truck every time we breathe, the consequence of this is that in time the physical body learns to use the respiratory muscles the wrong way, becomes addicted to adrenaline and then dysfunctional in some way. This is an abnormal response to survival, life and living.

Another normal response to pressure is when a person runs a speedy one hundred metres. The body reacts in much the same way. The same adrenaline based panic mechanism is fired off, the same feelings are felt. When the run is over, the body settles down naturally, the brain releases endorphins and the feelings of panic or stress subside, firstly, because we deliberately allow ourselves to relax and, secondly, because this is what we expect should happen.

There are many situations when the adrenaline rush is normal, the excitement and happiness felt when hearing good news, attending a happy event – marriage or an engagement party, winning a race, getting a new job, finding work after being out of work, passing examinations, or any excitement or danger of any kind that keeps us safe and happy.

So what happens if an individual is exposed to too many stresses, for example, prolonged unhappy or abusive relationships year after year and, one shock and trauma after another? The body goes into panic overload. It stays in a state of panic. The whole body is compromised and so too is our health.

If the nervous system is systematically sensitised to panic then any excitement good or bad will automatically trigger the adrenaline cycle and the associated symptoms and characteristics of Anxiety Syndrome. The adrenal glands do not know the difference between good and bad excitement and so the cycle continues.

Case History

A patient came to me and told me a very sad story. She was twenty-eight years old. She had lost five family members within two years and had been in a car accident herself.

By the time she came to me she said that she felt as if her life had a feeling of unreality, it was completely out of control and she felt numb. She was suffering from constipation, severe migraines; she lost her temper easily, had heart palpitations, hot and cold flushes, and felt detached from those around her.

As part of her search for the answer as to what was wrong with her, she had gone for counselling and was happy with the outcome. She said that she felt that she had dealt with most of her grief issues but said that she felt that there was still something wrong.

Before living through the traumas she was a normal healthy functional person.

After I explained to her what shock does to the nervous system she was able to identify with many of the physical, mental and emotional symptoms associated with Anxiety Syndrome. She was very relieved to know what was wrong.

She understood the theory of what had gone wrong, and said that she had noticed that she was breathing high and shallow in her chest and wondered why.

She worked really hard to get herself back on track by learning to breathe correctly and within a few weeks was back to her normal self.

notes

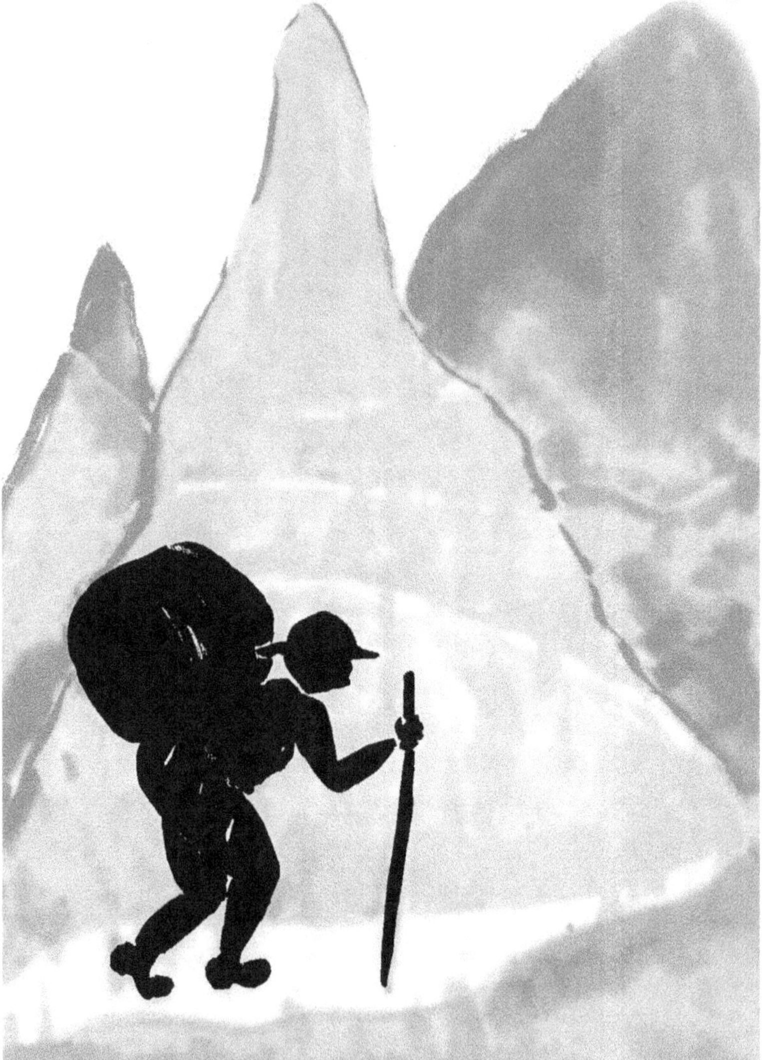

The longest of journeys begins with one small step.

The trek

Basically this story is about how I entered the portals of Depression. Why I stayed there so long, how I perpetuated my stay there, the diseases I suffered from during that time, my trek through the maze of misinformation and misdiagnosis of what was really wrong with me, and how, and where, I was when I stumbled upon a treatment.

The Trek itself began with a shock. My neck was affected. I went into shock, froze then panicked and for a few seconds thought I was going to die. Everything happened very fast and those few seconds changed my life forever.

> " ... I went into shock, froze then panicked, and for a few seconds thought I was going to die. "

I had always been in control of my life and my actions, whereas, from that time on, even though the shock passed instantly, as shocks do, the after effects lasted for years.

The initial shock sent me spiralling into post-traumatic stress. I began to suffer flashbacks about the incident and experienced nightmares, something I had never really experienced before. I felt disconnected from myself, others and, my surroundings and began suffering from the symptoms of multiple anxiety disorders. I began to live in fear. I began to fear fear itself.

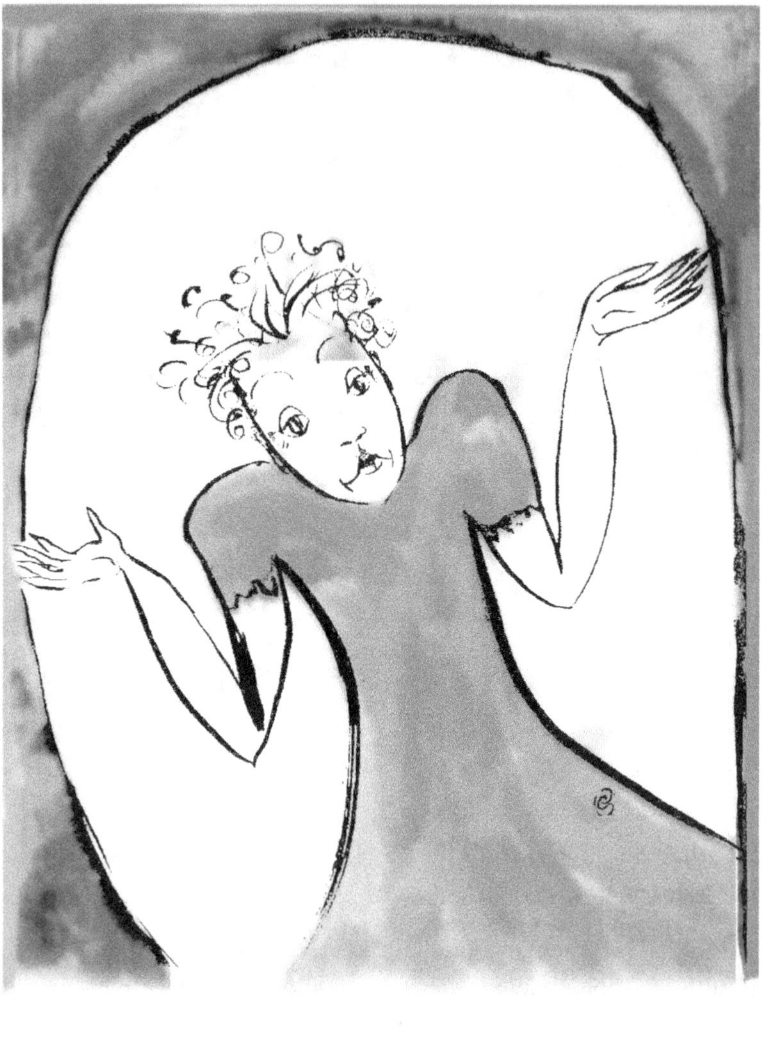

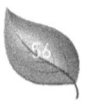

I was living inside a black cloud of fear...

I felt faintly sick and nauseated most of the time, dizzy and disoriented. I suffered heart palpitations together with shortness of breath, and breathed high and shallow in my chest. I always felt as though I could not get enough oxygen and worrying became a way of life. I did not worry only about every day issues but about everything past, present and future.

I could not sleep properly, if I did go to sleep I would wake up suddenly and not be able to go back to sleep, and I always woke up tired.

I was really into 'prevention is better than cure', and nearly ran myself ragged keeping my children 'safe'.

I seemed to have two minds. One that could think rationally and one that was on automatic and never stayed still long enough for me to have any peace, and my body followed suit - it was always on the move.

I was forever moving the furniture around, changing the layout of the garden, moving from one place to another, one house to another, one state to another or one country to another.

These symptoms caused my attitudes and behaviours to change, I knew I was normal and yet I knew that I was not normal. This reality is very frightening and gradually I started avoiding people, places and situations that made me feel anxious - in other words, I kept away from people, places and situations that triggered my symptoms.

I slowly and steadily became Socially Phobic and Agoraphobic and withdrew from living a normal interactive life. I found that I could not go up in lifts, down in parking areas, stand on the edge of a cliff or building without feeling 'funny' and, I could not ride on escalators.

I was living inside a black cloud of fear, I could see everyone and everything on the outside of my black cloud but I did not feel as though I was in any way part of, or connected to, what was 'out there.'

The 'Syndrome' affected my whole life.

From being totally in control of my life I was now feeling physically chaotic inside myself, I felt as though I had no control over my life any more, and began acting in ways that were foreign to me and to others.

I felt as though I had been another person before this time but I could not access her normal reactions to anything.

I felt as though I had to learn or relearn how to live, almost as if there were two of me, except that those two people could not reach each other, and therefore, could not work together to create one identity. I felt as though I was being pulled in two different directions at once. Maybe only people who have felt like this will know what I mean.

My learned normal and predictable reactions to things no longer happened as they always had and I began to live in fear, worrying about whether I would behave in an acceptable manner. Fear became a way of life for me. Instead of being in control of me, and my life, I now felt as though I was at the mercy of every whim and wish of those around me.

And so my frustration, anger and resentments grew, and it showed. I did not know this at the time, but have realised this since.

I now know that my primary driving force was fear, and that all through those years, instead of letting anyone see how frightened I really was, I would cover it up with bravado or anger. I never felt angry with anyone else, only with myself for not knowing what was wrong with me.

Many of my clients have shared with me the same fears. Like me, they have become really good actors. They too could 'put on a front, carry on and do their work', and because they could not get any answers as to why they felt as they did, they too learnt to hide their feelings, because, as they have said, "who would listen anyway?"

Family and friends just told us to pull ourselves together.

I can remember feeling really hurt when a close relative of mine said to me, angrily, "all you need to do is some exercise", the implication being that there was really nothing wrong, I just needed to lose weight and get fit. She was right. I was both overweight and unfit. However, because of the Syndrome, every time I did any exercise I would become even more tired.

> "All you need to do is some exercise, ... the implication being that there was really nothing wrong, ..."

Climbing up a short flight of stairs made me feel exhausted, out of energy and breathless. This was my constant dilemma, how could I walk, run, exercise or ride a bicycle for miles to lose weight and get fit when I could hardly lift one leg after the other because I was so tired and out of breath?

We anxious people know that there is something wrong. That is our greatest worry. We do every medical and non-medical test available to find out what is wrong, right through to counselling, both psychological and psychiatric, and each time come out with a clean bill of health and a list of past-unresolved issues we could look into.

We search into our own past personal history. We analyse to death our family histories looking for the answers. We try prescription drugs and, in many cases, non-prescription drugs and other chemicals.

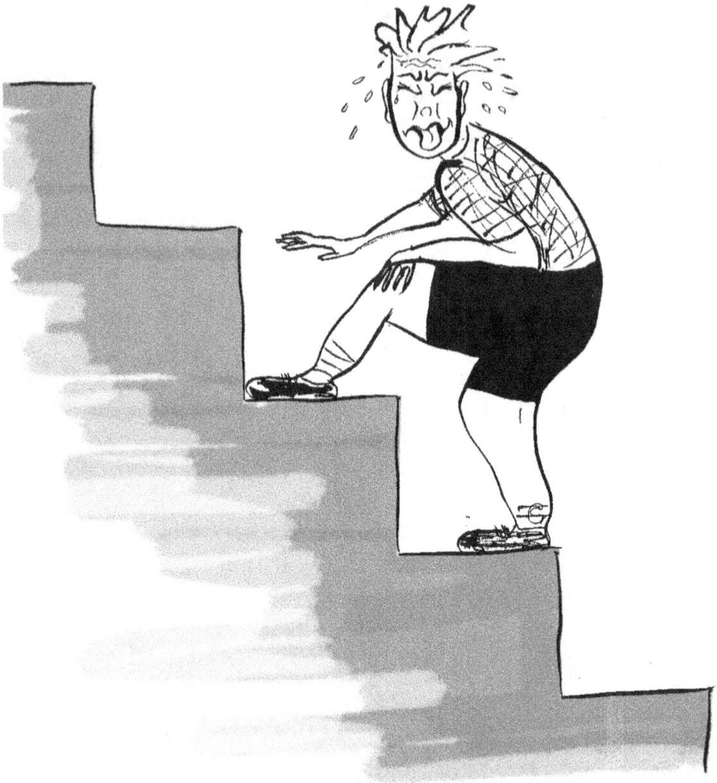

*Climbing up a short
flight of stairs makes us feel
tired, out of energy and breathless.*

We attend every self-help course available and, in fact, attend every course available to us, until we became course junkies.

We do Meditation, Tai Chi and Yoga, and try all types of religions and spiritual paths. Read books on every conceivable subject, but all to no avail, and all of this whilst still expecting to live reasonably productive lives.

For a while every new course or new idea got my adrenaline going and I felt good, but it never lasted. Afterwards, I would spiral down again and my search would continue. I knew that I had not yet found the answers I was looking for.

Like me, my clients knew that there was nothing wrong. They were normal, rational, logical, healthy people, but they also knew, as I did, that somehow, somewhere, something was wrong. Because of the fear element, thoughts like these escalate our feelings of anxiety and our search for the answers.

We processed (analysed) every thought that went through our heads. We knew that there was nothing wrong with our brains or our thinking. We knew that we could think rationally and objectively and use our commonsense to deal with life's normal pressures, but we also knew that something was wrong.

Over the years I went through the whole spectrum of medical problems that can mimic real medical diseases.

Chronic Fatigue Syndrome, constipation, diarrhoea, headaches, migraines, hyper/hypoglycaemia, upset stomachs, nausea, vomiting, wind, bloating and burning in the stomach, asthma, neck pain, shoulder pain and lower back pain, constantly swollen ankles. Suspected diabetes, thyroid problems and high blood pressure plagued me for twenty-five years. All these diseases coupled with expending the effort needed for day to day living, year in and year out, left me more exhausted than ever.

Everyone misdiagnosed my symptoms. I was told that I was having a nervous breakdown, that I was suffering Depression, that my iron levels needed boosting and that there was nothing wrong. I was told to go home and be a good wife and mother, and this I did time after time, each time making up my mind that I would get on with my life.

I was told that I had not resolved my 'many' past and present family issues when, in fact, I had actually analysed myself right into developing my own therapy, JETT, 'Johnson Emotional Trauma Therapy', a therapy which in the space of a few seconds releases those persistent still pictures, like 35mm slides, stored in the minds eye. The pictures always lurking just below the surface, the ones that would not go away and let me forget what had happened to me, pictures that held me in the imprint of the emotional shocks/traumas I had suffered. I did not see moving pictures inside my mind of what happened, only still pictures.

Release can come about in about thirty seconds as the picture disappears. Letting go of the emotional tags attached to the pictures can be really life changing. I always felt then, and still do now, if I use the therapy, as if a burden has lifted off my whole body. I feel lighter, my mind is clearer and the light seems brighter and objects around me seem clearer and more defined. It is a complete clearing.

It took me twenty-four years to sort this system of releasing emotional 'tags' out and I am much stronger now that I have de-traumatised myself from nearly every past major issue which was negatively affecting my life, but this did not stop my Anxiety Syndrome.

I still needed another key. That was to come. Within a year I had the answer I wanted – I found the Johnson (Breathing) Technique!

At times I was manic and full of adrenaline (high) energy and could do and achieve anything that I wanted to achieve, especially if I was helping other people or concentrating on doing something that took my mind off me, and my problems, such as studying. At other times I was depressed/down.

I now know that some of the Depression I felt was as a result of the normal natural balancing of the physical scales of energy.

Highs and lows are normal. If I drive myself to achieve and put myself under pressure to perform for any length of time, these days, I know I will have a quiet, down or depressed time following. So I give in and rest.

> " Highs and lows are normal. ... So I give in and rest. "

This, I believe, is a normal mechanism of energy balancing within the body. It allows the body time to recover so that it will be ready for the next set of demands that will be made upon it.

There is another 'down' side to Anxiety Syndrome. From some of the work I have done, I have found a connection between anxiety symptoms, characteristics and addictions.

Continuously feeling mental, physical and emotional anxiety symptoms will cause people to try to stop feeling their feelings by either 'drowning' them with alcohol, or 'hiding' them behind a smoke screen – cigarettes or drugs, for instance.

They are trying to stop feeling their feelings for a short time. However, as time passes and the feelings do not go, more and more alcohol is needed to keep the feelings submerged until alcohol takes over and addiction follows.

Smoking, on the other hand is a 'meditation stop', a way of calming the body down, giving it a rest from its feelings of stress if only for a few minutes. It is 'time out'. One of the reasons why we find it so difficult to give up smoking is because we have nothing else to put in its place to de-stress the body.

Using the Johnson (Breathing) Technique will help to calm the stress symptoms and enable you to start having the strength to give up your smoking habit. Take your time get the breathing technique right first.

Many addicts in the short term hide their anxiety symptoms by taking chemicals, however, in the long term, much greater damage is done and so they spiral further down into feelings of loss. Their behaviours and attitudes change, they lose their self-esteem, self worth, money, family, friends, homes and jobs and for many they lose 'self'. They completely lose their identity.

It could be that Anxiety Syndrome is an addiction in its own right. The body loves the adrenaline rush. I think the body becomes addicted to the chemical adrenaline and whether the 'high' is negative or positive the body will seek to have more of it.

My younger age group clients say that they love the adrenaline high that comes from bungy jumping and any other form of excitement but they hate the surge of unwanted adrenaline overdose at other times. Many of them know that adrenaline is the problem and are grateful to have a way of controlling their linked behaviours and attitudes especially in the areas of work, love and relationships. However, more and more young adults are coming to me to understand how they can break, for instance, their alcohol addiction.

When I say to them that they have 'learned' to be successful in their chosen career, however, if they started drinking when they were about fifteen, they have also 'learned' how to become an alcoholic. They are really dumbfounded and the usual comment is that no one has ever explained it to me like that before. They have practiced becoming an alcoholic for years. They then ask how do I change this, what do I do next? I always suggest they look at the adrenaline addiction first.

Many addictions can be linked to adrenaline. Alcohol, gambling, drugs, eating disorders, Anorexia-nervosa, Bulimia, smoking, sugar, chocolate, workaholics, perfectionism, exercising excessively (gym junkies), retail therapy, shopping, collecting anything obsessively, Obsessive Compulsive Disorders, (O.C.D.), SMS texting, computers and other addictions too numerous to mention here.

Adrenaline is the primary addiction. All other addictions are secondary to adrenaline. There is a saying about addictions. If you give up one addiction, another will take its place without us even realising what we are doing, however, if we can lessen the control adrenaline is having over our lives, it might follow that it will be possible to take control of our other addictions also. Much work needs to be done here on a long term basis to prove any of this. I have not had the time to take this further.

Stress is a modern day problem and is seen in our society in epidemic proportions. It can and does affect nearly every one of us at sometime in our lives - *stress* does not discriminate.

However, it is up to us to recognise our own needs, all of us breathe approximately fifteen times every minute of every day, it is so easy for each one of us to check what the physical body is doing. Are your shoulders raised, is there tension in your abdominal muscles, are you panic breathing do you feel stressed.

Ask yourself do you need to harness your adrenaline energy? If the answer is yes then do so by using the Johnson (Breathing) Technique.

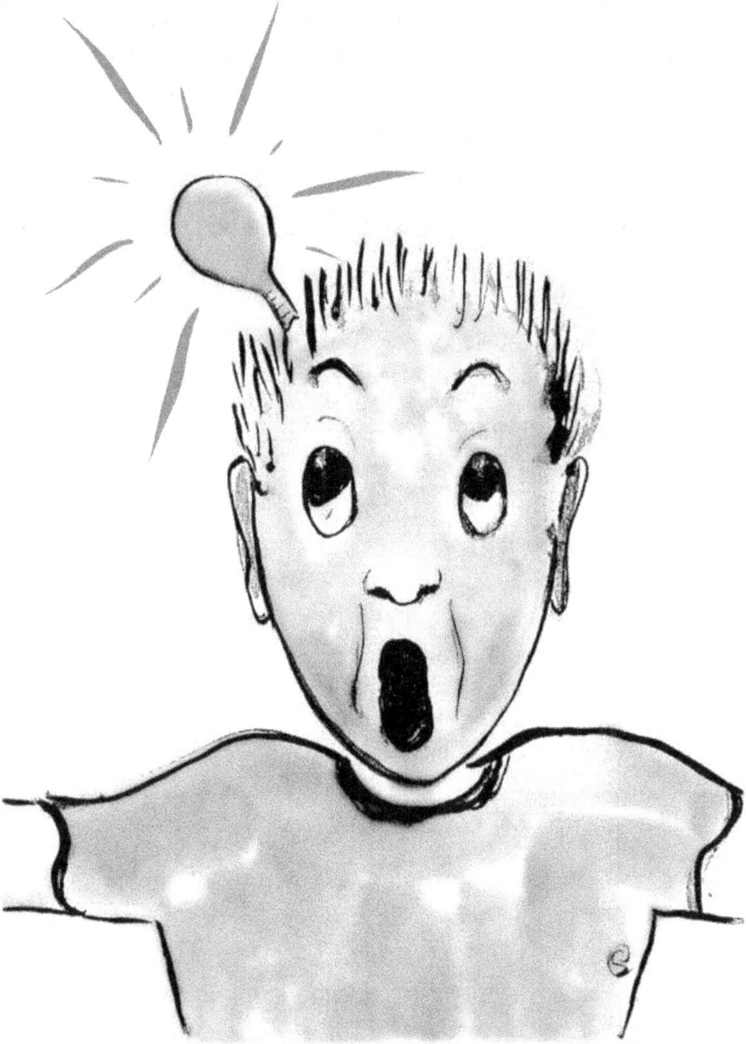

*Now I know what has been wrong
with me all my life!*

(Quotation from a young English Gentleman)

BINGO! it wasn't just me suffering!

My biggest challenge throughout all of this was not to be beaten I had to believe in myself. I felt sorry for myself and needed to keep reminding myself that there must be another way. Even though I knew I was not the initial catalyst for what happened to me, I also now knew that I was the one who was keeping my syndrome going.

I new I had to find a reason for being here and, a purpose.

I had the answer literally at my fingertip. What I had to do was remember to use my hands apply the Technique and retrain myself to technically breathe normally. If I did, my body automatically corrected the adrenaline flow and peace followed.

> " I had the answer literally at my fingertip. What I had to do was remember to use my hands ... "

For about two years I stayed 'stuck' in the shock of finding a way to heal myself and resisted dealing with my anxiety problem. I was in denial. After so many years suffering, I liked the comfort zone I was in. I did not really want to believe in the simplicity of the theory and Technique and, therefore, the efficiency of the treatment. I had found my reason and purpose but was resisting, both, shifting and healing.

I was pushed! After realising how many others were also suffering, enlightenment gradually dawned upon me and I decided to really do some work on myself. I had to prove that the Technique worked for me before I could effectively teach it to others. At last, here was something that gave me a reason for living, and a purpose, it was something I could do both for myself and for others, and it was so easy.

This book is written from both personal and professional experience. As a Naturopath and counsellor I can honestly say that the feeling of relief I felt when I found out what was wrong with me, is only surpassed when I see someone I am working with, begin to relax and feel peace within, sometimes, for the first time.

I see the same relief, amazement and euphoria reflected over and over again on the faces of my clients, it is the most rewarding and satisfying feeling a Practitioner can have.

They too have broken down in tears of relief. I have heard comments, such as, from a young Englishman, "I knew I had to come to the Gold Coast, Australia, even though it is only for three days. Now I know what has been wrong with me all my life. When I leave here I'll ring my Mum in England and tell her I'm okay. She's been so worried".

This young man was twenty-nine years old and had been a millionaire, but was forced in bankruptcy just before he left for the Gold Coast. He added I can do it again, I can make another million, but I could not fight this.

From an elderly, wealthy German gentleman, who had spent $10,000.00AUD, over the previous two years trying to find out why he was always sick. He just sat there looking stunned and said, "... and you charge me so little, I cannot believe it". Later when he heard how easy the Syndrome was to treat, he said with tears of relief in his eyes, "it is so simple. All I have to do is change my breathing."

Knowing what was wrong released him from his fear and the adrenaline rush and gave him the freedom to start taking control of his life again.

More recently a sixty year old son brought his eighty-four year old mother to see me, saying she feels dizzy all the time. He said she has been everywhere and no one can tell her what is wrong.

I asked her to show me what she does when she stands up. She stood up. As she did so she prepared herself, to cope with 'feeling dizzy', by taking a big full breath high into her chest and simultaneously pulled her abdominal muscles in. I saw at once what she was doing to cause the dizziness. I suggested she sit down again well back in the chair drop her shoulders down and let her abdominal muscles relax.

She immediately said I feel much better. After explaining to her what she was doing to herself and how she could change it, she said, with a giggle, "all I have to do, is it let it all hang out". She had never had a day's sickness in her life until she suffered a heart attack six months earlier, when her body went into shock. She said, "It *was* a great shock".

The biggest issue for all of us who suffer from Anxiety Syndrome is - control. We feel that we have little or no control over the symptoms and characteristics of anxiety and, therefore, have no control over our lives.

In order to keep the peace within our own bodies, we try to keep the peace around us, by forcing others to bend to our individual or collective will. We know that the only other alternative is to withdraw altogether, avoiding all people and situations that disturb us.

Believe me people with Anxiety Syndrome will do anything to keep the peace. If they don't, they feel as though they are losing control and going mad or insane.

They become over sensitive to light and sound. They want both the lights and the sound turned down even if the lights are not too bright or the sound too loud.

They appear to be rigid in attitude. They will not change their minds, move or give an inch in an argument, or, conversely they will be the opposite forever free flowing in thought, word and deed. They keep themselves and everyone around them moving in order to be in control of the situation, for example, house moves, career moves. Moving stops everyone from having/making any permanent long-lasting relationships so there is no need to learn social integration skills because, 'we will always move on'. They will be hopeless with money or control the purse strings rigidly. They will either spend everything or do the opposite and save/keep it all. Everything about anxiety is in extremes making it very easy to identify.

> " ... Everything about anxiety is in extremes making it very easy to identify. "

The other extreme of the always on the move cycle, is the anxious people who cannot cope with change of any kind and will stop everyone else from changing and moving. They will always have a good excuse as to why changing or moving should not happen.

We are often called 'control freaks'. However, most of us only want normal control over our lives. We want to keep the peace within ourselves. Most of us do not want to control others we just want to live normal happy functional lives ourselves.

What is not normal is the behaviour of the involuntary nervous system when it is continually impacted by prolonged stress, shocks/traumas and/or when it is under pressure to meet normal energy

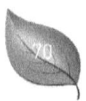

demands, for any length of time, after which it is not given enough time to recover. Energy becomes depleted and a general spiralling down begins causing acute, then chronic fatigue, weight loss/gain and feelings of being 'down' or depressed.

We bring this upon ourselves. Using our minds we force our physical bodies past the point of coping, and sickness is the response. The body is expressing its need through sickness. The message here is that it needs time to rest and heal - but when do we ever listen? The nervous system is the most important system in the body it needs 'time out' it needs time to calm down. Stop pumping adrenaline. Calm the nervous system down and let all the support systems, glands and organs go back to work.

Case History

Many years ago a friend of mine told me that she and her husband had reared three young children whilst running a seven-day a week business for fifteen years.

At the time I met her I was curious as to why she was in such good health. She was in her early sixties. She said that she believed that if she had not slept almost continuously for three months after selling the business, she would not be so healthy today.

She also said there were many times when she thought that she would never get off the bed. Gradually her body just recovered naturally from her prolonged stress. Her energy returned and twenty years on she is very healthy and active and has a new love in her life! She did add, however, that she still has a rest whenever her body tells her that she needs one.

notes

Trial, error and understanding

What happens to the nervous system? Why and how does the nervous system respond to prolonged stress and intermittent shock/trauma messages that are sent to it? What treatment is available?

I believe that the nervous system becomes sensitised to the continuing pressures of stress and trauma. The triggers, both known and unknown are received by the subconscious system causing the body to panic - to experience the fight, flight and fright, freeze response. Feelings of fear and anxiety escalate and our thinking, attitudes and behaviours change to cope.

> " ... Feelings of fear and anxiety escalate and our thinking, attitudes and behaviours change to cope. "

To explain this further, one needs to understand how the body works.

There are two systems in the body, the conscious, voluntary system and, the subconscious, involuntary system. The conscious, voluntary system - the thinking mind sends messages, thoughts, from the brain. These messages are picked up by the subconscious involuntary mind and nervous system, which then responds by acting appropriately.

Cell biologists' research shows that the subconscious mind is programmable. It has a mind of its own it is not controlled by the conscious mind. For example, once a person has learnt to drive a car, the whole procedure just becomes automatic. We do not have to think about how to drive the car, only about where we are going. We have programmed what to do into the subconscious system, it takes over and we drive automatically.

What is the cause and effect of Anxiety?

The subconscious mind controls all the internal systems and parts thereof in the physical body, the blinking eyes, lungs, beating of the heart, digestive system, stomach and bowel, kidneys, adrenal glands, reproductive system, etc. This subconscious mind does not think for itself, it is a conditioned mind it can be trained by the conscious mind to take on good habits, e.g. writing, or bad habits, e.g. technically breathing incorrectly.

Consciously we cannot alter the action of the subconscious system permanently, e.g. the action of the eyes, or the beating of the heart. However, and this is the key I was searching for, there is a bridge between the two systems, the technical action of breathing. It is this action we can be change.

We inherit a nervous system. How we breathe is ours alone. Breathing is the one thing we can change and the reason why anxiety problems are not inherited. Using the respiratory muscles the wrong way all the time causes us to run on adrenaline, therefore, the cause of stress and anxiety is a technical problem in the physical body connected to the way we breathe. The function of the body and mind is chemically changed if we use the upper and lower abdominal respiratory muscles of the body incorrectly.

We attempt to fill up our lungs by lifting our shoulders, expanding our chests, raising our shoulders and pulling our abdominal muscles in, so that we can take in as much air as possible. This is exactly the action that is taken when a person wants to jump out of the way of, e.g. a speeding vehicle. This is the fight, flight response. Every time we take this action the message is sent to the rest of the body that the fight, flight or fright, freeze response needs to be activated. The body is flooded with both oxygen and adrenaline and conditioning begins - a bad habit is learned, the body learns to breathe using the respiratory muscles the wrong way and adrenaline addiction takes over, the body loves adrenaline and will always seek more of it.

Rather than having too little oxygen we have too much and we are, at the same time, helping ourselves to become addicted to the chemical adrenaline and like any addiction the body learns to want more.

If we pull our abdominal muscles in and breathe high in the chest often enough, the nervous system will systematically learn to release adrenaline. This then becomes a habit. Adrenaline can be triggered at any time by technically pulling the abdominal muscles in, standing up straight, whilst pulling our shoulders up and back helps to cement this pattern.

Therefore, activating the body to technically breathe correctly is the key to lowering adrenaline, controlling weight, stress and anxiety levels. Breathing is the only link between the voluntary and involuntary systems and is the only action that we can alter.

I have noticed, and you will have noticed also that people under stress often sigh. They lift their shoulders to help the initial intake of oxygen and then continue with shallow/high in the chest breathing, almost like panting – panic breathing. They are encouraging their adrenaline addiction by breathing like this.

This is not the normal or correct way for the body to breathe except in a stressful situation. If one continues to breathe like this for any length of time – hours, days, weeks, or even years, then the symptoms conditioned into the nervous system over this time will become a habit, just like hand writing, or driving a car. The symptoms are caused by a learned bad habit.

> **"** ... the nervous system is painstakingly conditioned over time to automatically run on adrenaline. ... **"**

We do not have to think about how to write – manoeuvre the pen. When we are writing a letter, we only need to concentrate on the words we are writing not how to use the pen. We have already painstakingly learnt how to write. We do not have to think about how to drive a car because we have painstakingly learnt how to drive. Once we have learnt to drive we automatically drive, all we have to do is think about where we are going.

Exactly the same happens with anxiety symptoms. Breathe high and shallow in the chest, and pull your abdominal muscles in and the nervous system is painstakingly conditioned over time to automatically run on adrenaline. Worry often enough and the conditioning continues.

Breathing correctly will balance the gaseous exchange in the lungs, drop the adrenaline level in the blood and re-energise the organs, glands and systems. We need to become aware of our symptoms and retrain ourselves to activate the body to breathe correctly.

Physically helping the body to harness the chemical adrenaline by reversing its breathing pattern from high and shallow breathing in the chest to lower abdominal, (below the waistline), breathing, will help the body return to its normal natural peaceful state, all the internal systems will begin to work properly and weight control is possible.

notes

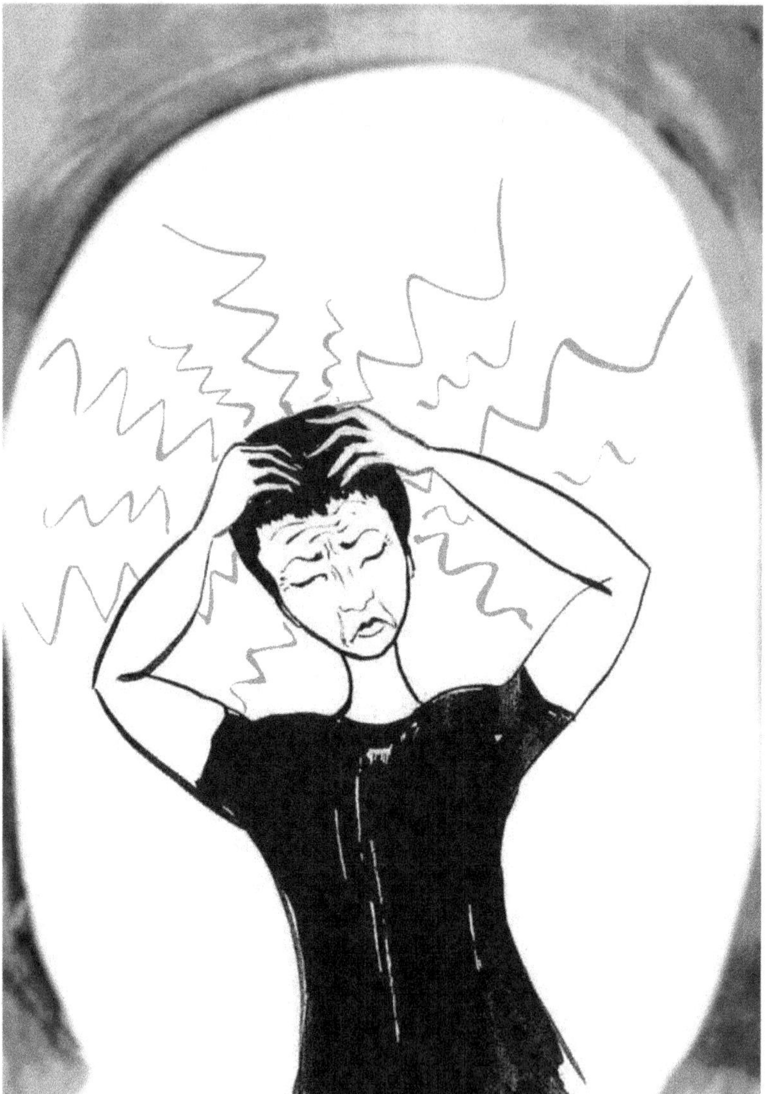

Common physical symptoms anxiety mimics.

Disease symptoms of adrenaline addiction

When helping clients to understand what Anxiety Syndrome is all about, I ask them if they have had diabetic, thyroid, urine and blood tests, etc, before I follow through with showing them that their various symptoms could be related to anxiety and the adrenaline pattern. The reason for this is because anxiety symptoms can mimic other diseases.

Correct diagnosis is critical when treating Anxiety Syndrome and I encourage my patients to read about their symptoms. They need to relate to what I am talking about. I also encourage them to interact with me about what is happening right now, because, if after previously being tested for everything and nothing is wrong, then more than likely Anxiety Syndrome and adrenaline addiction is the problem.

> **" Correct diagnosis is critical when treating Anxiety Syndrome ... "**

- Headaches - migraines

- Diarrhoea

- Constipation

- Back/shoulder/neck pain – lactic acid and adrenaline go hand in hand, therefore, after running on adrenaline there will be a build up of lactic acid, this exaggerates painful conditions

- Wind/bloating – stomach and bowel

- Burning stomach, acid, reflux

- Eating disorders and other addictions

- Insomnia - or altered sleep patterns

- Acute and Chronic Fatigue Syndrome

- Incontinence – passing water (urine) more often than necessary

- Asthma (nervous) – can be stress related – use the breathing technique. (Do not stop taking any medication without your Doctors consent)

- Hyper excitability, hyperactivity

- A.D.D./A.D.H.D.

- Hyper/hypoglycaemia – high and low energy

- Behaviour changes, e.g. fanatical behaviour appears to be adrenaline charged, and so too is bad or aggressive behaviour.

- Mood swings

- Depression

- Tinnitus - noises in the ear

- Post-natal Depression for men and women

- Hypertension and high and/or low blood pressure

- Thyroid problems

- Toxaemia/fluid retention

- Immune system is less effective because it slows down during stressful times and sickness follows, e.g. phlegm, mucus problems, influenza, colds, viruses, sinus and sore throats and, always feeling under the weather and catching every little thing that comes along

- Food allergies – many are related to stress because the digestive system does not work properly when the body is in panic, not enough digestive enzymes are produced. The energy normally required for the digestive system is needed elsewhere. Ulcers. Skin problems, rashes, eczema, acne

- Irritable Bowel Syndrome (IBS), (colon) – correct identification of the adrenaline rush, plus technically breathing correctly will aid in treating and curing this problem, however, perseverance, persistence and patience are needed because it takes a long time, but it is worth the effort

- High cholesterol, heart attack and strokes are all, I believe, connected to stress. However, always ask you doctor for advice before starting anything new

- Weight gain, weight loss or no control over weight.

81

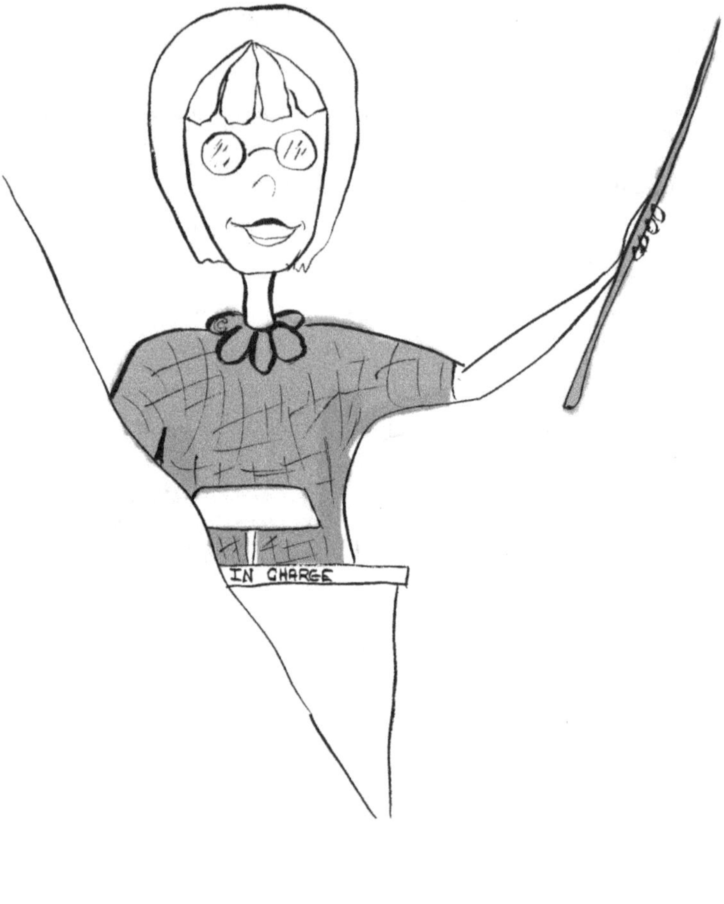

Regaining self control!

Control at last

Five years ago, I attended an addictions counselling course in the beautiful Southern Highland of New South Wales, Australia.

This was a very stressful time for me. My son had just had a serious accident in one of the mines in Mt. Isa. I did not know how serious the accident was until I returned home, three months and many thousands of kilometres later. However, lack of knowledge and distance did not stop me from worrying constantly about him, and this coupled with the stress of the course I was doing, caused my own Anxiety Syndrome to escalate out of all proportion.

> " ... distance did not stop me from worrying constantly ... "

First of all, I hated doing examinations - many anxious people panic at examination time. We had an examination every Monday morning. Secondly, I had never even heard of the Twelve Step program, whereas everyone else attending the course had some background knowledge of this. I spent the whole course in catch up mode.

At one stage the pressure became too much for me and I took myself off to a medical doctor. She took my blood pressure and told me there and then that I should give up the course and go home or she would put me in hospital until my blood pressure came down.

I said, "No". I needed to complete the course and went back to work.

I do not recommend here that others follow my action. However, by trusting my own judgement I did the right thing.

During the week that it took for me to get over the shock of how high my blood pressure was, the most amazing thing happened.

I found out how to control my Anxiety Syndrome.

Feeling tired one afternoon, I decided to lie down before dinner and rest my weary body. I was feeling very sorry for myself. I was a long way from my home; I had a very sick son, a migraine and severe pains in my lower abdominal area. I felt as though I wanted to be sick and my ankles were severely swollen.

As I lay on my back holding my lower abdominal (gut) muscles with my hands I suddenly realised that all the pressure was seeping out of my body and that my mind had stopped racing. What was happening, I asked myself?

Gradually my migraine became only a headache. My ankles stayed the same until the next day but the pains in my abdomen disappeared and I was able to go to dinner. I found, for the first time in ages, that I was really hungry. And, all I wanted was good healthy food, no rubbish or junk food.

Fortunately, when the changes inside my physical body occurred, I had the presence of mind to note down exactly what I was doing. During the next week I practised the same routine at every free opportunity.

For the first time in years I found that I could stay calm if I practised what I had observed. This was a wonderful feeling. Instead of feeling cold all the time, I began to be filled with peace, warmth and calmness.

I felt really happy and enjoyed the rest of the course and managed to complete it successfully.

Slowly my blood pressure returned to normal. At last I knew how to stop the chaos.

The speed of my rehabilitation was exhilarating, (adrenaline, of course) but, oh, how I enjoyed it! I sped from doing the Johnson (Breathing) Technique lying down, to sitting up, to standing up and, control was mine at last. Gradually I began to control my inner self and consequently my life.

I graduated, but more importantly I left the course with the knowledge I really needed.

In hindsight, as I have said before, isn't it wonderful, I can see that the basically strong and resilient person that I am had to be brought to my knees before healing could come about?

I had to become really ill before I could find out what was wrong. This I now understand and accept, although, I hope that I never have to walk that path again. The loss of quality of life, pain and suffering was almost more that I could live through.

However, if what I went through can change the life of one person for the better, then I will know that I did make a 'difference' after all. I will know that it was worth it, not just for me, but for another also.

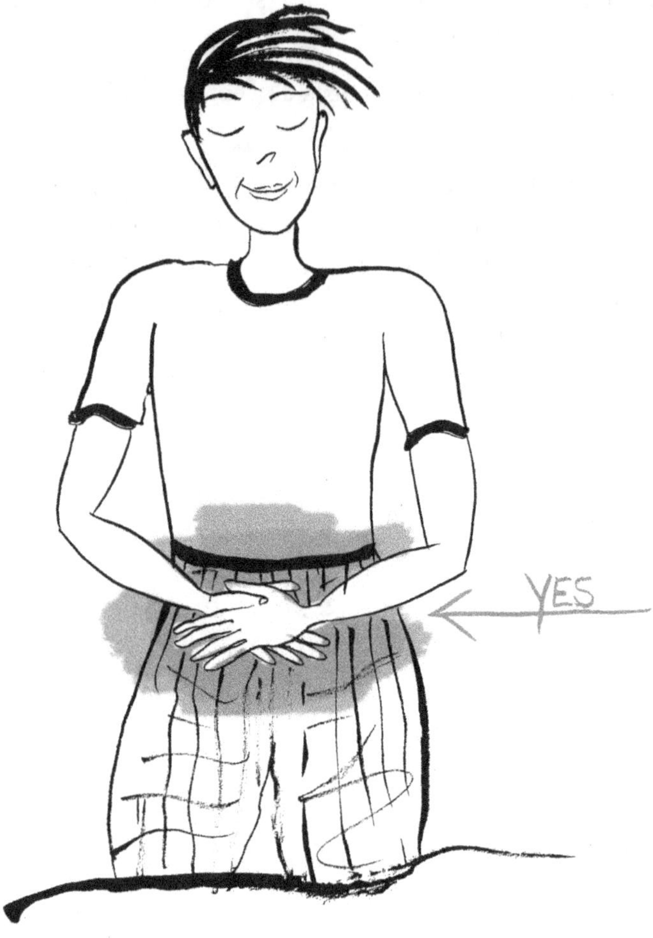

YES

Place your hands one on top of the other - palm to the back of the other hand - three finger-widths below the belly button.

Johnson (breathing) technique

BEFORE STARTING THIS EXERCISE, PLEASE READ THE DIRECTIONS

We were born breathing the right way and the physical body will easily go back to that way of breathing if we let our learned conditioning go. It - the physical body - is not made to run on adrenaline all the time, *we* have programmed it to run on adrenaline and *we* can change the patterning.

For the purpose of the exercise the lower abdominal muscles are sometimes called the 'gut', or the power centre.

This Technique can be used at any time - lying down, (supine or prone), sitting or standing, but the easiest way is to lie down on your back, on a firm flat surface, use a pillow under your head only if you need one, otherwise, no pillow. This enables the body to breathe easily, particularly when gravity intervenes and there is no pressure on the abdominal muscles. However, the most difficult position to master is the sitting position.

> " ... we have programmed it (the body) to run on adrenaline and we can change the patterning. "

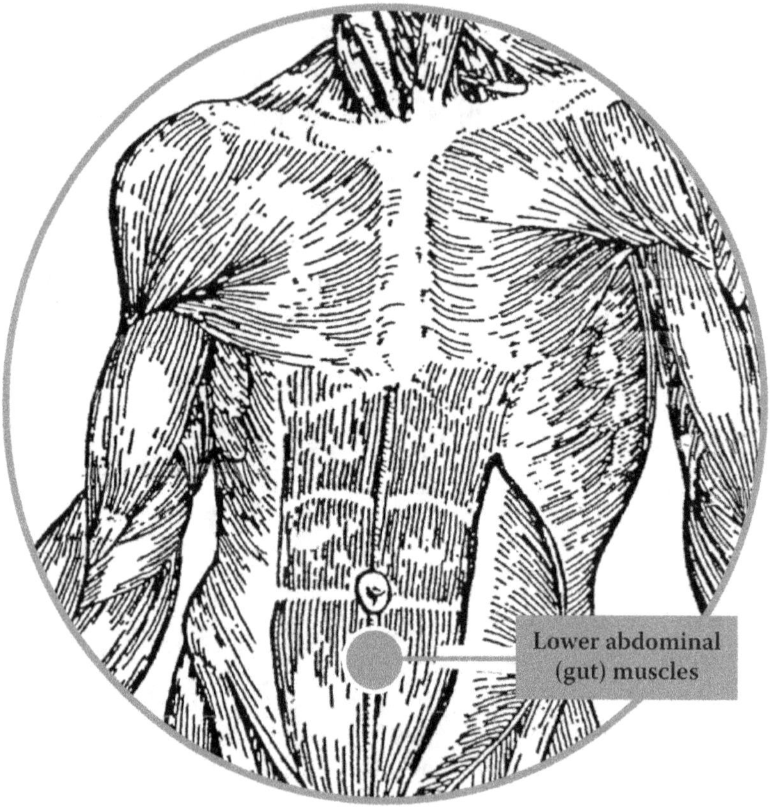

Lower abdominal
(gut) muscles

If your feet do not reach the ground when you sit on a chair – men, women and children – use a step. Always putting pressure on your abdominal muscles as you hold your feet off the ground can cause physical stress and anxiety.

Step 1
Sitting position

Sit on a straight-backed chair, with your feet flat on the ground and your spine straight. Make sure your buttocks are firmly resting against the chair back. Support your lower back above the hips, at the waistline, with a small cushion if necessary. Relax and sit evenly and balanced on your buttocks. Do not lean back, lean slightly forward.

Allow your stomach and abdominal muscles to fall outwards/forwards towards your thighs and allow your shoulders to drop down and forward, just relax them, in other words, slouch. If you slouch your shoulders and abdominal muscles by relaxing them you are not altering the position of the spine, therefore, the spine which has natural curves in it is still 'straight' only the rest of you is relaxed. Many of you will feel the tension go out of your neck, shoulders and back if you can relax these muscles, immediately releasing some neck, shoulder and back pain.

Step 2

Check yourself at the beginning and at the end of the exercise to know your level of success.

Assess your level of comfort. Do you feel comfortable or uncomfortable sitting in a slouched position and is your mind running on and on?

The answer is usually yes to at least one of the above. Mostly it is yes to both of the above.

At the end of the exercise check yourself again. By then the adrenaline level should have dropped the body feels more comfortable sitting in a slouched position and the mind has stopped running on.

Checking yourself like this is your way of knowing if you are successful. You should feel a lot calmer, if not much more tired. Because of your adrenaline addiction, your body *is* tired it has been running flat out with a fast moving truck chasing it for years.

Step 3

The Technique

Using either hand, find your power centre by measuring three finger-widths below the belly button (umbilicus). Place your pointer/index finger on the lower edge of the belly button. Then place the next two fingers close together, beside the pointer/index finger. Fingers should be straight, and hand flat against the abdominal muscles.

When you have done this place the centre of the other hand, (centre palm), against the third finger of the first hand. Leave the second hand there, withdraw the underneath hand and place it on top of the second hand and rest the palm on the back of the other hand, just li the 'yes' picture.

The thumbs are near the level of the belly button. The power centre should be in the centre of the hands and that is where the focus of the mind is when doing the exercise. Do not focus on the thumbs and the belly button, if you do, the Technique will not work properly. The focus for both mind and hands is on the power centre.

Step 4

Remember to slouch. Check the tension in your abdominal muscles you may find that you have, out of habit, pulled them in again. Let them go, let them sag – relax, slouch. As you do this you will feel yourself begin to relax. We all tense up so take your time, feel some of the tension/stress seep out of your body, your muscles need to learn how to work properly again. This is a very important key, and the whole point of the reprogramming exercise.

You have been holding the abdominal muscles in all your life and now they are resisting. They do not know how to relax. It's a habit.

Step 5

Observe your own rhythm of breathing, you may find that you are breathing fast, high in the chest, very shallow, or are even holding your breath. Relax become aware of the rhythm and pattern of your breathing only. This exercise has nothing to do with the lungs it is a technical problem concerning the action of the respiratory muscles above and below the belly button (umbilicus) at the waistline.

Step 6

Starting the exercise

Always start by taking a breath in – inhale, then, as you breathe out-exhale, use your hands to push, gently, the lower abdominal muscles in towards the spine. Push them in towards the spine as the air is breathed out, almost as if you are pushing the air out from the power centre, (gut), rather than from the lungs alone.

At the same time as the hands are pushing the air out use your internal physical strength to pull the muscles under the hands in towards the spine, then let the muscles go so that the body can breathe in again. Remember to focus on the middle of the hands - on the power centre. Do not roll the hands, push straight in towards the spine then relax both the muscles and the pressure of your hands together. Do not remove your hands.

Step 7

On your next 'in' breath release the pressure of your hands on the 'gut' muscles and relax the muscles, feel them relax forward, almost as if the air is going right down into them. Physically <u>push</u> the muscles out from the inside, away from the spine to help the natural action. This is a muscle hand coordination exercise, a Cognitive Behaviour Technique (CBT).

Continue practicing for a few more breaths as often as possible until you feel familiar with this new breathing pattern. Do not pressure yourself and become distressed especially if you are a perfectionist, if you have read and understood the theory you will be processing how to use the Technique on a subconscious level. Learn first how to slouch, the rest will follow. Then do the exercise every time you find yourself pulling in your stomach muscles, lifting your shoulders, or holding your breath.

We are all aware that pulling the stomach in will improve our appearance, however, we also do it when we are stressed, not realising that this affects the function of the physical body. Technically both actions cause adrenaline to run. The body does not know the difference.

The body will resist this new way of breathing for two reasons, one, it loves the chemical adrenaline and two, the body has previously learned a bad habit which it wants to hang on to.

Become aware of your breathing, become aware of your body and use the Technique constantly for **_six weeks_** to re educate and re program the physical body and mind to take up its normal breathing pattern. Gradually retrain your body by learning to become 'aware' of the tension in your 'gut' (lower abdominal muscles), and shoulders. Once you have become more 'aware' of your own tension areas and levels you are well on your way to living in a mentally and physically calmer state.

When doing the exercise, you are exaggerating the action of the lower abdominal muscles.

We think we need more oxygen. In reality we need to have a better balance between oxygen and carbon dioxide and the other gases in the lungs. Using the respiratory muscles the wrong way causes the imbalance. It is this mistaken thinking about oxygen and the following action that is part of the problem.

Breaking old habits, ideas and conditionings

In this exercise you do not alter the normal flow of your breathing. Do not follow the pattern of breathing in through your nose or out through your mouth. For those of you, who have used a visual meditation technique, do not think about the colour of your breath or which side of your nose you are breathing through. Given time the body finds its own natural balance.

Most importantly of all do not count. In other words, take no notice of the upper half of your body, (above the belly button) except to observe your rhythm of breathing.

Your lungs have been breathing the same way since you were born and do not need any help doing their work. There is plenty of room inside the ribs for the lungs to breathe without you helping them by either lifting your shoulders or puffing out your chest.

This exercise has nothing to do with the core centre of the body. The full concentration of the exercise is on the power centre and the 'gut' where the hands are placed not on controlling the breathing or imagining where the 'core' centre is. The lower abdominal muscles at the power centre are the controlling muscles.

It is not a mental problem. The only part the mind plays in this is in 'directing', controlling the hands and, therefore, the lower abdominal (gut) muscles to work properly.

A black belt Martial Arts person explained to me that the reason this breathing exercise works is because the power centre of the body is located exactly three finger widths below the belly button.

Focusing the mind and hands on the power centre will centre the energy of the body, giving the body a chance to relax so that it can release all feelings of anxiety and stress. When focusing the mind on what your hands and gut are doing, you will drop the adrenaline and not be able to think about anything else. Therefore, the Technique works for all forms of nervous tension in mind and body. Using the lower respiratory muscles correctly causes the diaphragm to work together with the lungs.

We cause our own anxiety. How many times have you been told to stand up straight, pull your stomach in and pull your shoulders back?

We think we are a fat society. How many times have you pulled your 'fat' stomach in to flatten it?

Standing up straight, pulling your shoulders back and your stomach in is the signal for flight and flight, the body recognises this action and responds by releasing adrenaline. We have all been told to do this. If we put on to much weight we try to make ourselves look slimmer by holding our stomachs in and it is this action which defeats what we really want, i.e., to lose weight, it also effectively teaches the body to want more adrenaline and the adrenaline addiction continues. We are doing this to ourselves.

As I have already written. I do believe, however, that changing your breathing alone is not enough if you want to lose weight. A healthy diet and exercise programme helps and is very important in the long term for maintaining optimum health.

For best results, learn to breathe correctly first. Bring peace into your life and balance your energy. Build your physical energy up by giving the adrenal glands a bit of a rest.

> " For best results, learn to breathe correctly first. Bring peace into your life and balance your energy... "

At the same time start correcting your food intake – smaller portions, increase the 'good for you' foods and lessen the 'bad for you' foods, we all know what they are. Then chew your food properly. Digestion starts in the mouth, the stomach is not meant to do all the digesting. When you feel a bit stronger and have a bit more energy from eating 'good for you foods', start very slowly an exercise program. It is always recommended that you have a health check with you health practitioner before starting any new program.

The Technique is both a cognitive behaviour technique and a distraction method.

Concentrating ones mind on the hands when breathing naturally, keeps the mind focused and slows the speeding thought patterns down, whilst at the same time calming the whole nervous system.

Teaching the body to physically use the respiratory muscles correctly when breathing will help you reverse panic breathing and thinking, both the mind and the body are calmed at the same time by relearning how to do something perfectly normal and natural, breathe.

The action of placing the hands on the abdomen at the same time as concentrating on the breathing is a mental anchor and works really well for most people, however, for those who need an extra anchor to reinforce the changes you want to make, I include here another anchor.

After breathing in and out twice with your hands on your 'gut', on the next 'in' breath, without moving your chest, take a deeper breath by pushing your abdominal muscles further out from the spine. Exaggerate the action. Hold your breath for the count of six, and then breathe 'out', as you do so, push the muscles in with your hands and continue with the normal exercise. Do this only once in any exercise cycle.

> " These anchors and hand actions send a clear message to the brain ... "

It does not matter whether you are standing, sitting or lying face up or face down on a bed, only hold your breath once. If you do it more that once the body does not recognise it as an anchor and will think it is learning another breathing technique

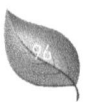

These anchors and hand actions send a clear message to the brain and the system generally that you are making changes, and gradually over a period of time the system responds more quickly and begins to settle down almost as quickly as it escalates into panic. In future, if you have practiced enough, as soon as you place your hands on the power centre, the body will respond and start using the respiratory muscles correctly.

You have retrained it to relax on command. The body will resist at first because it does not like being forced to change an ingrained pattern, nor does it want to let its adrenaline addiction go.

To prove that the body knows what to do, lie down on your back on a flat surface, (preferably without a pillow), and observe for yourself where your body moves, when you breathe in and out.

If you give yourself enough time you will notice that your chest stops moving as you continue breathing and your abdominal muscles take over, they begin to rise up when inhaling and sink down again when exhaling. This is the normal action of breathing.

What we do when we panic is normal also. However, what we do the rest of the time, if we allow the body to run on adrenaline and panic, is not normal, it is just a bad habit. If ones nervous system is sensitised to stress then this bad breathing habit perpetuates stress and anxiety making our lives totally miserable.

If you cannot make your hands and arms work properly sitting and standing, then lie down, the only problem with doing it this way is that you will have to learn to use your hands at a later date.

In my opinion there is no permanent cure for Anxiety Syndrome because once we are conditioned to any good or bad habit it is there to stay. Adrenaline is normal and can activate every time we breathe if our posture is incorrect.

We breathe fifteen times every minute, therefore, it is possible to always be running on adrenaline, however, it is also possible to gradually break the hold adrenaline addiction has on the body and mind by following the guidelines laid out in this book.

I consider that we are 'in recovery', because even though we can control it, it will return. It is like any other chemical addiction, except that this chemical is inside the body and it is called adrenaline.

As time passes, healing comes about and our quality of life improves. With understanding, practice and persistence we can learn to 'harness' our own adrenaline energy. This will give us more control over our health and, therefore, our lives.

This system, theory and Technique, has worked for me and thousands of others. I wish you every success.

Conclusion

Since I started practising what I am preaching, my life has definitely taken a turn for the better and last year was an exciting year for me.

Realising how many other people are suffering from the same problems I decided to do something about helping them if I could.

I searched long and hard to find ways of reaching others so that they too could learn to overcome their anxiety states. I thought of going into schools. I thought of visiting various self help groups but for personal reasons I could not go too far afield.

> " I searched long and hard to find ways of reaching others so that they too could learn to overcome their anxiety states. "

However, two ideas did evolve out of my brainstorming, one was to run anxiety identification groups, and the other was to run seminars for anyone who wanted to know how to diagnose and treat Anxiety Syndrome.

Both ideas were very well received and I duly set about arranging to bring a group of people with Anxiety Syndrome together so that they could identify with each other what happens to them when they become anxious.

At the same time I suggested to other Naturopaths and healers that I would start running seminars, and teach them how to recognise and treat nervous problems.

The identity group for anxiety sufferers was very successful.

These were not group therapy sessions, where patients worked through their issues but rather group sessions where they could all talk about how anxiety was affecting them.

Anxious people are by nature very conservative, however, once the participants realised that others needed to hear their stories, so that they too could identify, they were very happy to share and help each other. By sharing, they quickly realised that they could help others in the same way that they needed help

The Anxiety seminars were also successful. As a health care provider I know that it is very easy to look at individual diseases and treat the symptoms rather than the cause, however, understanding what happens to the nervous system when it is stressed, helps enormously to correctly diagnose and treat.

Before I finish writing about Anxiety Syndrome and how it nearly destroyed my life I would like to share with you an example of a time when the Johnson (Breathing) Technique saved me from great embarrassment.

Case History - one of my own.

The last seminar I ran in 1999 was an interesting experience.

As I walked into the room carrying my books and notes, I was overcome by the worst panic attack ever. The adrenaline rushed through my body and my legs went to jelly.

I was wearing a red suit. My face went red, my eyes were glittering, my breathing was high and shallow and my heart was thumping. I was shaking like a leaf and I thought to myself - well here goes, let's test my theory.

I walked to the nearest chair, sat down, put my books down on the desk and physically forced my body to breathe correctly.

In three breaths my system returned to normal and - I just knew it worked.

My body settled down and I was able to enjoy myself teaching people to do something that really works and doing something myself that I really enjoy doing - teaching.

Before I learnt how to control my anxiety I could never stand up in public and either interact with a group or give a seminar comfortably. However, now as I begin to lecture, I breathe correctly and settle myself down.

I no longer want to feel that adrenaline rush through my body except when it is for fun, happiness or excitement. No more red faces, pounding heart and headaches and legs going to jelly for me.

notes

Commonly asked Questions and Answers

Question

What are the most important things we need to remember?

Answer.

1. When practicing, always make your hands move in and out or the body/mind connection will not learn to respond automatically at a later date when you place your hands on the lower abdominals/ respiratory muscles.

2. Practice as often as possible.

3. When you stand up, or move suddenly from a relaxed position to, e.g. answer the telephone, hold you breathe for a split second deep down in the lower abdominal area. Then, as you move, release the air immediately, so that your breathing continues. This will stop you from feeling dizzy when you stand up or move suddenly.

Question

How do you tell the difference between mental illness and multiple anxiety disorders of the nervous system?

Answer I encourage everyone who is breathing incorrectly to correct their breathing first. If clients are able to discipline themselves into breathing correctly, after I show them what to do, often their symptoms will become less. If they cannot cope with this new way of breathing then there may be other reasons and medical advice should be sought for further diagnosis.

Question

Do you interfere with prescribed drug taking?

Answer No. I refer patients to a medical doctor who will help them bring their drug dose down if they want to do this. I leave this assessment entirely up to the doctor.

Question

Do some patients need to stay on their drugs, e.g. Anti-depressants?

Answer Yes. They have a chemical imbalance, and, as insulin dependent diabetics need and use insulin to enable them to have quality of life, so too do anti-depressants offer quality of life to patients with some forms of anxiety.

Question

Is self-diagnosis a good idea?

Answer   No. Health care practitioners are trained to diagnose. What the general public needs to do is find a health care practitioner, either medical or non-medical who will listen to what they are really saying.

Take a book to your health care practitioner, such as this book and tell them that you think you are suffering from Anxiety Syndrome. Ask them to do the appropriate tests to confirm your opinion and if they will not listen to you, find another health care practitioner who will listen. One, who knows about adrenaline, will listen to you and help you.

Question

Do I need to breathe through my nose to do this exercise?

Answer   Yes and no. Do not think about breathing, the body and lungs know what to do they know how to breathe without your help. Concentrate on what your hands have to do to stay in tune with your natural normal breathing rhythm, there is no need to think about your nose and mouth.

Question

Does Meditation, Tai Chi, Yoga and Pilates help?

Answer Yes and no. In the long term they do help because they all work on a subtle level. In the short term we need to learn to breathe correctly all the time to keep our nervous systems calm and not just when we are practising the disciplines. We breathe approximately fifteen times every minute.

Generally speaking, when we finish practising any of the above the first thing we do is stand up. As we stand up we take a big deep breath, almost like a sigh, high into the chest, lifting the shoulders as we do so, and it is this action which defeats what we have just been practising. Immediately the physical body is thrown back into the same way of 'panic' breathing and the Syndrome continues.

N.B. As you stand up after these exercises, hold you breathe down in the abdominal muscles for, as we say a split second, this will stop both the oxygen and the adrenaline rush and also stops you from feeling dizzy.

Question

Do we inherit multiple anxiety disorders?

Answer In my opinion no. We all inherit a nervous system that is ours to do with as we want – we can breathe to keep it calm or we can breathe to make it run on adrenaline, this is our choice. However, if we have a parent who role models panic/anxiety or a phobia about spiders, for example, then more than likely we will take on the same fear and model the same behaviour.

Question

How often do we need to practice the Technique?

Answer As often as possible for the first six weeks, especially before going to sleep and after waking up in the morning. Practice as often as you can during the day or night. Notice when you shoulders and abdominal muscles are tense and when you feel stressed. Once you have practiced the Technique and you know it is right it only takes three breaths for the body to spontaneously calm down. Once you know what to do and do it, you can remove the fear of panic, anxiety and any other symptoms of adrenaline addiction.

To be effective and get lasting results you need to be very consistent with your practice using your hands for the first six weeks so that you lock in the new conditioning. By then you will be aware of your breathing habits and will pull yourself up when you find that you are tense. Practice, perseverance and patience will get the best results. Use the hands, push them in and out – make them work, otherwise the body/mind connection will not listen and learn to respond spontaneously. Eventually when you place your hands on the gut you will automatically take a deep breath and start breathing correctly.

People suffering Anxiety Syndrome are typically driven by adrenaline and do not have much patience, therefore, they need to recognise this as part of their problem and break the pattern. There is no quick fix.

Question

How long do we need to practice?

Answer In the beginning, practice for a short time only. Getting the discipline right, at first, is more important than length of time. The more you practice the easier it will get. However, as you progress your physical body will respond to your hand action by calming down more quickly after about three breaths. If it is not working for you, you are not concentrating or practicing correctly. Some people learn more quickly than others. Some people take a week to learn to, slouch, drop the shoulders and let the abdominal muscles relax they are so conditioned to holding the body in 'tension'.

Question

When do we use the exercise as a calming response?

Answer When you can do the exercise properly learn to recognise your anxiety symptoms/triggers and do the breathing. You should begin to calm down in a few minutes. Although sometimes much longer is needed because you are not focusing your mind on your hands and what they are doing.

Question

Are there any side affects to this exercise?

Answer Yes. When you have done the breathing correctly you may experience a slight dizziness just behind the eyes. This is not hyperventilation.

I think this happens because the chemical balance in the blood changes, e.g. less oxygen and adrenaline, and the brain responds by releasing endorphins to calm the body.

If you feel dizzy, stop doing the 'technical' breathing and sit breathing as naturally as possible - do not panic. Keep your hands placed on your gut and keep your mind there also – the dizziness will go. Do no take a big breath up in your chest, this will cause the adrenaline to suddenly escalate and hyperventilation may follow. Hyperventilation is connected to panic and adrenaline, and oxygen and carbon dioxide.

Within a short time a feeling of calm seeps down over the body and release from anxiety symptoms follows. You will then notice that your mind has stopped racing, your symptoms have calmed down and you are breathing normally with abdominal muscles moving in and out and relaxed.

If you have bowel/colon or stomach problems, do the exercise lying down on your back at first. Do not force your lower abdominal muscles. Just rest your hands on the power centre and your mind will automatically focus there. Over a period of time if you can practice the breathing and get it right, you may find that some of your problems begin to disappear anyway.

Question

What are other stressful situations?

Answer Stressful situations are many and varied – driving in heavy traffic when you are running late, having your blood pressure taken, being given an injection when you hate needles, and going to the dentist.

When your spouses/partners, in-laws, parents or children make it very plain that they are critical of you, or disapprove of you in some way.

Examinations – school, university or medical examinations.

Before and after the birth of a child, both parents get very stressed so both should try to breathe normally, so that they can relax and enjoy the experience with the new baby and, with each other.

Breathe to calm yourself down before public speaking and when you wake up suddenly during the night and cannot go back to sleep.

Breathe normally in a lift or aeroplane, and also if you are scared of spiders, snakes or leaving the house and the taps or iron on, etc.

When any situation, place or person upsets you, calm yourself and your mind down by breathing correctly. Stop panic breathing, stop the adrenaline rush and technically make your body calm down. Practice using your hands until you can direct your body about what to do, at will.

There are hundreds of stressful situations. Make your own lists. Be gentle with yourself. Know what panic is all about and that the fear will pass as it always does.

PRACTICAL EXERCISES

Head one list 'My Own Internal Triggers'. Notice when you are breathing incorrectly. Write down your mental, physical and emotional thoughts, feelings and sensations and also when you know that you behaviour and attitudes change.

Start noticing when you are holding tension in your shoulders and abdominal muscles – relax them.

Observe your mind, when you are worrying and cannot turn your mind off. Ask yourself what is it you are worrying about? Is it important?

If you are worrying about something in the past, it has already happened and you cannot change it, if you are worrying about the future, it may not happen so you may as well live happily in the here and now and stop worrying.

Head the other list, *'External Triggers'*. Include in it the places, people and situations that trigger your anxiety.

write your list in the space below if you prefer

_____

_____

_____

_____

_____

_____

_____

_____

_____

_____

_____

_____

_____

notes

Testimonials and case histories

ANXIETY - ANOREXIA NERVOSA

For four years I was suffering from anxiety and I was unaware of it. From doctor to doctor, tests after test, and many visits to the hospital due to dehydration everything showed up clear physically.

I was healthy, but why was I still feeling the way I was. I was not able to stomach any food or had any appetite to eat, continuously vomiting all the time due to this I lost a whole heap of weight which had led me to the beginning stages of anorexia due to my anxiety.

> **" ...and many visits to the hospital due to dehydration, everything showed up clear physically...** **"**

Finally, I was diagnosed with a general anxiety disorder by a doctor whom I was recommended to see, and I was able to work around the anxiety and fix this. I thank God I was sent to this doctor, as I was going crazy and so was my family. A simple diagnosis was missed many times.

This has changed my life, now I have much more understanding of what I was going through, why I lost so much weight and now my family has gained knowledge and understanding of anxiety. I thank my family for all their love, support, patience and understanding through all of this. This experience has taught me so much in life most importantly self acceptance within yourself, however, we are not alone.

Helen's breathing technique assisted me when I was down, when I felt an attack coming and when I am feeling anxious. Now I breathe normally through my gut and find that I am much more relaxed and sustain happier life, knowing how to effectively treat myself when ever I feel anxious, so thank you Helen.

Regards JK

P.S.   *JK was given my book by her Aunty. She did the diagnosis of anorexia herself and worked out how to do the breathing with the help of her family. She is back to her normal weight, has stopped the fluctuations of weight she was experiencing and is much happier. She does not live anywhere near me, however, I have since met her and her family and we are all very happy with the results. Helen.*

IRRITABLE BOWEL SYNDROME

I saw Helen Johnson for the first time in January 1997. I had severe Irritable Bowel Syndrome (I.B.S.). I had suffered with this problem for fifty-two years and she was my last hope. My life was totally miserable - I have lived in South East Queensland all my life and knew where every toilet was.

After seeing her on a regular basis for about a year I went on my first overseas holiday to New Zealand with two friends at Christmas 1997, and thoroughly enjoyed myself.

I had never had a live-in relationship to that time or been on an overseas trip.

I have worked full-time all my working life but I was very stressed and tired because of my problem.

You do need persistence and perseverance in finding an answer and then someone to lead you in the right direction.

D.L.

P.S.   *Persistence and perseverance is very important in treating this problem, however, I now know that doing the exercise on a consistent basis will bring about good results in a much shorter time than is mentioned above. I too have more experience and knowledge. Helen.*

A TESTAMENT OF MY "NERVOUS" LIFE

November 2001

The following testament is a condensed 30 year story of how an undiagnosed nervous disorder has severely afflicted my life. It also states how in the three months since the disorder has been diagnosed that my quality of life has rapidly improved as I continue to practice what Helen Johnson had explained and shown to me.

At a very early age in my childhood it was obvious to my parents that something was 'not right'. From about one year old they had noticed that my speech patterns were not developing normally. The sounds of the words I was trying to say were so garbled that no-one could understand what I was saying. I was four to five years old at the time that my younger sister became my interpreter; she somehow managed to decipher my talking.

Being the concerned & loving parents that my mother and father were, I was taken to several 'childhood experts'. Nearly all of them thought that my abnormal speech patterns were a sign of brain damage/mental illness. But, having an above average intelligence and showing no symptoms of any cerebral disorder I was thrown into the 'too hard basket'. No-one knew how to deal with someone who didn't fit into any standard medical category.

One so-called 'childhood expert' determined that I was suffering from deafness, so much so that I was put into a hearing impaired school. I only lasted a week there after being the only pupil in the school's playground to hear and point out an airplane flying overhead. That diagnosis was very quickly discredited and discarded.

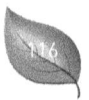

I eventually attended a 'normal' kindergarten. The head teacher there thought I was developing too slowly to be ready for primary school, so I was kept back there for a second year. However, halfway through the year my parents pulled me out as I was showing signs of boredom and discontent.

At age six and a half years I commenced primary school. I proved to be very proficient in the classroom although my speech patterns made life in the schoolyard a misery at times. Finding that solitude was the best way to avoid being treated as a social outcast was a pattern I continued right through into adulthood. I avoided school team sports, hardly every associated with a group of children and never had any friends at my place.

> " ... Finding that solitude was the best way to avoid ... "

I later had school-based speech therapy sessions which slightly improved my speech patterns. I was still speaking much faster than normal which made me barely understandable to most people. The only comfort I had was the fact that in the classroom I was consistently at or very close to the top of the class in various subjects, both at primary and high school level. It was my silent way of saying 'I am not stupid'. Something all the teachers I had knew to be true as well as me being very studious and very well behaved during class.

My social life as a teenager and adult has been virtually non-existent. I did not interact as freely with other students as they did with each other. I never had a girlfriend, a group of mates I could go out with or a person that I could call a close friend. I could detect that while some people did like me my speech patterns made them perceive that

I was 'not quite normal', and therefore kept their distance from me. The fact that social situations (like hotels, parties, etc.) make me so nervous that I literally become nauseous, clammy and uncomfortable reinforced my view that I was not able to have an enjoyable social life.

Job interviews were also a very difficult event to have self-control over. My speech patterns as well as severe nervousness had ensured that my employment prospects remained close to zero. Despite possessing a university degree and several other qualifications no employer-run interview had resulted in a Job, no matter how well suited I was to the position on offer.

As an adult I was starting to suffer from severe mood swings, feeling 'high as a kite' then so depressed that I wanted to completely shut myself from the rest of the world. I often wished that there was a dark closet I could lock myself in for as long as I wanted to, so that no-one would need to see me suffer from my internal torment. Even after gaining a permanent employment position, these mood swings persisted for no apparent reason.

Energy swings also became apparent with me suffering regular acute fatigue sessions. These made me so tired that I felt that my eyes were going to fall our & than I would spend many hours sleeping. Trying to relax and relieve the tension in my body was something I could not do. I regularly had severe painful cramps in my abdomen region. Again, I did not know the reason for all of it occurring.

My self-confidence has been very low nearly all my life. I did not feel that I would ever be regarded as '100% normal' by the society I live in. But just when I concluded that this and the above afflictions were to be with me for the rest of my days Helen Johnson came into my world and destroyed that assumption forever.

While describing the overactive nervous disorder to me, it was as if Helen Johnson knew me intimately. Consequent sessions with her

have given me the tools to bring the disorder under control. The chief tool is that of learning to breathe from the lower abdomen, something I was not previously doing.

In the three months since the first session my mood swings have moderated so much that I no longer suffer severe depression. The tension in my body and the pains in my abdomen have largely disappeared. Acute fatigue sessions have also become nearly a distant memory. But most importantly, my speech patterns have slowed down and improved so much already that even my parents are noticing a marked difference.

I am slowly starting to realise that I am a normal 31-year-old Australian male and can be readily accepted as just that (without the stigma attached with having a-speech impairment). I have recently been inside a hotel or two and not been nervous at all about it. I have enjoyed having a beer without fearing that I could become addicted to alcohol. People are not asking me to repeat myself when I say something as often as before.

My self-confidence is starting to rise as I teach more of the true me, one that has been held back for ages by the disorder. I have long felt that an elastic band was tied round my waist. Doing its best to pull me backwards while I was doing my best just to hold my ground let alone move forward. Thanks to the therapy and support Helen Johnson has given me I am slowly unravelling the elastic band and moving in the right direction, at long last.

D.A.

P.S. This young man had a really bad stuttering problem which improved very quickly. Helen.

MY NERVOUS LIFE

A Mother's Perspective

From an early age I knew there was something 'not quite right' with our son. A series of traumatic events happened during his early years, which well could have contributed to his disorder. These events included a near drowning and being in a household with a grandfather that was insensitive to him.

After taking him to various doctors, childhood specialists, etc. no true explanation was ever reached. He didn't speak often and when he did we could not understand him. The way he was understood was when his younger sister interpreted for him. When we took him for visits to other people's homes he would not get out of the car. We would leave him in there until he was eventually ready to come in on his own accord.

He was kept back a year in kindergarten but by September of the second year we took him away as he was totally bored. It was painfully obvious that he was highly intelligent and kindergarten was no longer enough for him.

During his school years he was constantly picked on by other children, mostly boys. The girls seemed to love him however and they interpreted his speech for him also. He attended speech therapist sessions during his primary school years but to no avail.

At high school I thought things would improve as he was by then mixing with older children. But things did not change. He still had no close friends and never had anyone to out house, which I thought was odd. But I thought his home was a haven for him away from the outside world. He excelled at school, was always a top pupil academically but was certainly a social outcast.

I thought things would improve when he worked at various jobs since leaving high school, thinking he would then make friends but he just seemed to become more withdrawn. Even when he went to university I still felt that things have not improved. My heart went out to him because I saw him as a very lonely young man. I wondered what else I could possible do for him because I would have done anything to help him.

He eventually moved out of our home after finally getting full time work. I kept calling him every week to 'check up on him' as I knew he had depression spells. One day in late August he rang me in a very excited state and said 'Mum, I think this lady knows what's wrong with me'. I told him to be careful because I knew how vulnerable he was and did not want anyone else to hurt him.

He saw Helen a few days later and within weeks there was a marked difference in his outlook on life, self-confidence and his dealings with me. When she told him that because he hadn't crawled as a baby that it contributed to his problem we all immediately got on the floor and crawled with him.

He showed me the breathing exercise that Helen had showed him to do in order to relax his nervous system. I do not go to sleep very easily so one night in desperation I tried the breathing exercise Helen had taught my son. The exercise worked straight away and I was asleep almost immediately.

Helen has been like a miracle to our son and to us and we are very grateful for her time and patience in her dealings with our son.

S.A

P.S.   *I questioned the fact that he did not crawl as a baby, however, I do not know for sure that this has anything to do with the development of speech patterns. Helen.*

STRESS PROBLEMS

I live in Bundaberg, Queensland.

My family and I have been using the Breathing Technique that Helen Johnson has taught us for a few years now and it has been a Godsend, it has rescued us on many occasions through Panic attacks, and stress problems.

I will not go into them all now, as there are too many of them.   If it was not for the Breathing Technique Helen taught us I do not know where or if I would be here now.

I even showed it to a friend at golf one day, as she was having trouble breathing and she thanked me, she later said, 'it has made a great difference in her life'.

The breathing helps you take control of yourself again when you think you are going to die or choke.

The Breathing Technique helped me and my family get through my Mother's four months of sickness and her death.

I thank Helen for giving us the breath of life to go on with.

L.W.

P.S I look forward to reading your book, Helen.

IDENTIFYING THE PROBLEMS

During my water polo career I have always succumbed to the enormous pressure that exists when training and competing at national and international levels. This pressure or anxiety plays an important part in any athleteís preparation.

However, I could not deal with the pressure and stresses placed upon me.

When I first became aware that the situation was not normal was at an international level. I was in New Zealand away from home and in a team I barely knew and who relied on my skills heavily. My team showed no signs of distress so I spoke to my coach about me feelings. The only reply was that it was just the jitters and its normal. 'Normal' is not finding it hard to breathe nor is it something that makes you feel

> " ... it was just the jitters and it's normal. Normal is not finding it hard to breathe ... "

so scared you have to escape to the toilet only to lock yourself in it so nobody can see you or talk tactics. This is not normal

Finally, from many encounters with this terrible emotional fear I confided in Helen Johnson. We identified the problems, planned future strategies and I was shown this unique breathing technique. With this new aid I no longer felt any further anxiety leading up to or during competition at any level. The breathing technique proved not only beneficial to my mental health but also to my sporting career as my development as a player improved dramatically.

This special technique not only has helped my sporting career but also in my education. Every year 12 student feels under pressure with the numerous assignments and exams placed upon them.

The beginning of term three I was ready to quit. I had had enough of everything, but by concentrating and maintaining the breathing technique the pressure evaporates. I then have the ability to focus on what needed to be done. I completed year 12 and received better than the OP I had wished for.

I believe that without this breathing technique I would not handle any stress placed upon me and also have never completed any of my major life goals.

K.P.

TESTIMONIAL OF HELEN JOHNSON

I found Helen through my partners mother. I was lucky I had people around me who cared enough to help me find her.

At the time I went to Helen I had been through a lot. I was suffering constant nausea, particularly at night, with shortness of breath from breathing too high in my chest and taking short sharp breaths, plus persistent diarrhoea.

I had this ever present feeling of pending doom, like there was something seriously wrong with me and I would stop breathing or die of something horrid. I was still working in a very demanding job, and felt like this everyday at work. I lost a fair amount of weight and felt like I'd 'lost' myself in the process too.

My first session with Helen was one of realisation, but there was reluctance to accept my illness, as I thought it was a weakness in me, but I realise now it was due to a lack of understanding and acceptance.

Helen enabled my partner, Tony, to be-present at my first visit, which helped tremendously. I wanted him to try to understand a little, so we could deal with things better, together. I called it an illness because of the physical symptoms.

I suffered from Anxiety, but week by week, Helen pulled me back a little further each time. She helped me understand what was going on with me physically and how I could deal with it, enabling me to gain more control each time. Breathing and controlling your thoughts is the key. You have to make yourself do it but once you have, you relax and start breathing steadily and feeling normal again.

Helen told me to find a book about nerves that was published in the early 60's. It was excellent, even though sometimes hard to read because of my association with it, that is, it made me remember the awful times when I was suffering acute Anxiety. Although the book was written some time ago, I could very easily understand it and relate to it. The most I got from the book was what Helen was guiding me to do, which was to stop fighting the symptoms, accept them and let time pass.

Prior to Helen, I was offered all types of explanations from other Doctors of whom some were on the right track, but there was never any follow up or the satisfaction I received from my visits with her. She helped me become aware of my triggers that cause Anxiety, which can sometimes be quite bizarre, but they are my bizarre triggers, no one else's.

This does not mean that no one else has suffered like me, as I began to realise from the group sessions I participated in with Helen and others. The group allowed me to identify with others and no longer feel alone. It helped that Helen suffers from Anxiety too and was strong in her counselling, giving me the ability to find strength in myself. You can 'cloud' the symptoms with drugs and denial, but I wanted to know how I ended up with Anxiety, and if I got to the state I was in without any artificial substances, then I could certainly get to where I am now without using them.

I did leave the Coast (where Helen is) for over a year and early on had a few bad nights suffering pains in my chest, was shallow breathing and had diarrhoea. I just kept remembering how Helen taught me to deal with the situation and with the support of my partner I came through, them those awful nights.

I gradually got better over time, i.e. 'I let time pass' and now I'm OK with the fact that I will never actually be cured of Anxiety. But I am healing more and more as days go by. I do see symptoms of Anxiety in other people now and if they are approachable, I tell them of Helen's work. I just hope the medical profession become more attuned in diagnosing Anxiety and refer them to people with Helen's expertise. She is my 'Healer', and my friend too.

L.W.

DEAR HELEN

I'm writing this to thank you for the work you have done for me and my family.

If only I'd known years ago that all I had to do was learn to breathe properly.

My life is more peaceful, my energy level is better and I can now go on long walks and my weight is going down.

As you know I'm Aboriginal and I would like to offer other Aboriginal people the help you have given me and my family.

I hope we can organize this.

R.N.

P.S. I'm walking 12 kilometres a day now that I can breathe properly.

CHRONIC FATIGUE SYNDROME

I am just so beside myself with excitement. I simply HAD to write to you immediately after our phone call.

As we discussed, after reading your book and after a major relapse, from 3 years of being virtually bed-ridden with Chronic Fatigue, I began your deep breathing method... instead of the more shallow type of breathing we seem to do in our modern day stress laden and sedentary age.

Within 1 hour I felt 50% better and within 2 hours I actually got up, had a bath and washed by hair (something I am rarely able to do with Chronic Fatigue). Then back to bed for more breathing... I haven't stop breathing since, & it is NO exaggeration to say that from the time of those very first 2 hours, that I started you deep breathing method I have experienced ABSOLUTELY NO pain or previous symptoms of my illness! (Apart from the general fatigue).

This is a complete turnaround for me! ñ going from CRIPPLING fatigue & nerve-wracking headaches, neck-aches & back-aches, queasiness, nausea, stomach aches and constant vomiting... sleeplessness, major digestive problems & chronic depression.

I also suffered a complete mental & nervous breakdown within the first year of going down, (becoming ill) along with nervous body jerks, muscle spasms & twitches, hyper-sensitivity to light & sound (from which I could not have survived without my mouldable ear plugs, & the mere sound of a passing car, barking dog or slamming door could send me into a frenzy of nervousness, anxiety & shaking).

I have since discovered that the paralysis, convulsions & neurological problems were caused by my (unwitting) exposure to white-ant treatment...

I have the dreaded Epstein Barr virus which keeps on ëhaving a partyí because of all the chemicals & heavy metal in my body, so it appears that although stress is considered to be the real trigger in this illness, it is so irritatingly complex with many other factors involved.

But what really amazes me is that despite so many different & varied symptoms associated with Chronic Fatigue, your technique of deep breathing into the bottom part of ñ or whole lung, has such a SPECTACULAR effect on them ALL...

And so, I guess, my job now is, simply, to 'spread the gospel' of the miraculous healing power of correct deep breathing, & if by any chance my story can help or enlighten others & perhaps prevent them from developing this most diabolical illness, then all my efforts & suffering may have been worthwhile after all. For in this modern age of stress, chemicals & environmental pollution this illness is rife & on the move. It is, exactly as my Chronic Fatigue brochure describes it, "absolutely devastating, debilitating & of immense & profound suffering".

So thank you Helen, from the bottom of my heart for finally awakening me to the simply miraculous healing power that lay locked within my own body - my very own God-given "Breath of Life"...

S.W.

P.S.   *I did not meet the author of this letter she lives thousands of kilometres from where I live. Her testimonial is many pages; this is an extract from her original letter. Her nineteen-year-old daughter bought the book from me and took it home to her Mother. S.W. did all the work on her own and spoke to me by telephone only after she had begun to heal. Helen.*

PANIC ATTACKS

Helen Johnson's Breathing Technique has helped me stabilise my life and my thinking. Over the years I have suffered from panic attacks which I could not identify. I did not realise that the shortness of breath, inability to sit still and the strange wish to flee or get away were all symptoms of panic.

After facing the consequences of a poor business decision which threatened to destroy a lifetime's work, my mental state was delicate. I faced a breakdown which was uncontrollable. I could not eat, sleep or leave the house. I constantly cried and dry reached. I was afraid. I was afraid of the telephone (dreading every time it rang) and could not get out of bed. I was on medication to help me face the day. The medical fraternity at large lacked understanding. Only one doctor showed understanding and explained that I was not alone, but could not provide me with help other than medication.

I did become stronger with the help of my husband and I managed to take myself off the medication. But I could not control or understand why I was continually in a state of fear. The vomiting attacks and crying would often be triggered by the simplest confrontation.

I finally found and confided in Helen Johnson about the uncontrollable fears and continuous worry I face every day. Helen taught me to understand these feelings and use breathing to control and alleviate my distress.

I can now calm down and sleep at night. If I feel my pulse racing and my breathing shorten, especially at night when the fear of life and where I am headed invades my thought and attacks me, I can use her technique and peace and harmony befall me and I am relaxed.

My thoughts and ideas are clear. I am studying at university externally now. I have the confidence to do so. I now realise that I had been avoiding making the decision to restart and upgrade my studies for nearly 20 years, despite wanting to – I was afraid to take the step.

Through Helen's technique I am able to study and achieve consistent marks of distinction.

I have been so inspired by this sensible and simple technique that I have started to introduce it to my class of 10 – 13 year olds. I teach several children with learning difficulties as well as two with behaviour problems controlled by medication.

We started using the breathing technique as part of our drama class and relaxation exercises. Initially some children could not lie still and concentrate. However, as we progressed and tried the technique regularly most children began to relax and concentrate.

Leading up to introducing the children to the breathing – this child had been destructive, violent and disruptive. After the session he remained calm, polite and in control for four days. As a strategy to relieve tension or curb deteriorating behaviour within our classroom we now at the first sign or hint of trouble take the children as a class through the breathing technique.

Our children are far calmer and relaxed. We laugh a lot and I believe the children now have a valuable strategy that can help them remain calm, focused and adjusted throughout life. I have recommended to several parents that their child would benefit from a consultation with Helen and her personal advice and assistance, especially the invaluable breathing technique.

L.R.

THE KITE

One day whilst attending my craft market stall, the kite I was using for demonstration purposes became entangled in a tree. My husband decided he would have to cut the line as he could not free it and asked me to follow the kite and collect it when it landed.

I chased the kite across a busy road and followed the path it had taken. I discovered it had landed at the top of a four-storey building and was hanging over the edge of the roof. To reach the kite and retrieve it I had to ascent an open spiral staircase.

Having suffered from terrible fear of heights for a number of years, I stood and wondered how on earth I was going to make my way up to retrieve it. I thought of the breathing technique that Helen had taught me and taking a deep breath I just gripped the rail of the staircase and went up one step at a time.

When I had retrieved the kite, I suddenly realised I now had to descend the stairs, which was even more difficult as I was now able to look down and see the ground. I stood there for a few minutes and told myself, "You can do this just take it one step at a time as you did when you climbed the stairs".

Taking deep breaths again, I finally made it to the ground; I had actually achieved something I had not been able to do for a number of years, thanks to Helens breathing technique.

J.H.

P.S. *This lady was in her sixties when this happened to her. She really did conquer her fear and understood how some of her other phobias, flying and crossing bridges in a car could also be conquered by applying the 'Technique'. Helen*

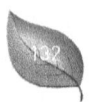

notes

notes

notes

notes

notes

.